# ARTRITIS COOKBOOK

## For newly diagnosed

Nourishing recipe and anti-inflammatory diet guide to alleviate arthritis discomfort and promote joint health

ANGELIA FRANKLIN, RD.

# Table of Contents

Copyright (c) 2023 ALLISON JACOB

# Introduction

Living with arthritis can be a daily challenge, affecting not only our joints but also our overall well-being. For those navigating the path of arthritis, understanding how to manage this condition is crucial. And one essential aspect of that management is diet.

Welcome to "Cookbook for Patients with Arthritis." This book is designed to be a culinary companion on your journey towards alleviating the discomfort and embracing a healthier, more enjoyable life despite arthritis. Within these pages, you'll find not only a treasure trove of flavorful and nutritious recipes but also a wealth of information on how diet can play a pivotal role in managing arthritis.

Arthritis is a complex condition, with various forms and degrees of severity, but one common thread among patients is the quest for relief. This cookbook is not a replacement for medical advice or treatment but rather a tool to help you make informed dietary choices that may complement your existing arthritis management plan.

In the chapters that follow, we'll delve into the world of arthritis-friendly cuisine, exploring ingredients known for their anti-inflammatory properties, practical tips for an arthritis-friendly kitchen, and, most importantly, a collection of delectable recipes designed to be gentle on your joints yet bursting with flavor.

Our goal is simple: to empower you to take charge of your diet in a way that not only supports your overall health but also adds joy to your daily meals. Whether you've been recently diagnosed or have been living with arthritis for years, there's something here for everyone—nourishing breakfasts, comforting soups, vibrant salads, satisfying main dishes, and even delightful desserts for those special treat days.

You'll also find guidance on creating meal plans, a grocery shopping guide, and useful cooking tips tailored to make your culinary journey smoother and more enjoyable.

Arthritis may be a part of your life, but it doesn't define your entire existence. With the right approach to diet and lifestyle, you can find relief, enhance your well-being, and savor the simple pleasures of food. Let's embark on this culinary adventure together, one delicious and arthritis-friendly recipe at a time.

So, don your apron, sharpen those knives, and let's create dishes that soothe both body and soul. Here's to a future filled with flavorful, arthritis-friendly meals and a life lived with more comfort, joy, and culinary delight.

Let's get cooking!

# Understanding Arthritis

# What is Arthritis?

Arthritis is a common medical condition that involves inflammation of one or more joints in the body. It is not a single disease but rather a term used to describe a group of more than 100 different types of joint disorders. The most prevalent form of arthritis is osteoarthritis, but others include rheumatoid arthritis, gout, psoriatic arthritis, and juvenile idiopathic arthritis, among many others.

Key Characteristics of Arthritis:

Inflammation: Arthritis is characterized by inflammation within the affected joints. Inflammation is the body's natural response to injury or infection and typically involves swelling, redness, warmth, and pain.

Joint Pain: One of the hallmark symptoms of arthritis is joint pain. This pain can vary in intensity and may be constant or intermittent.

Stiffness: Arthritis often leads to joint stiffness, particularly in the morning or after periods of inactivity. This can make it challenging to move the affected joints.

Reduced Range of Motion: As arthritis progresses, it can lead to a decreased range of motion in the affected joints. This can impact a person's ability to perform everyday tasks.

Joint Damage: Over time, chronic inflammation in the joints can result in damage to the cartilage, bone, and surrounding tissues. This can lead to deformities and joint instability.

Types of Arthritis: There are various types of arthritis, each with its own underlying causes and characteristics. For example, osteoarthritis is often associated with wear and tear on the joints, while rheumatoid arthritis is an autoimmune condition where the body's immune system mistakenly attacks healthy joint tissues.

Causes and Risk Factors:

The causes of arthritis can vary depending on the specific type, but some common risk factors and causes include:

Age: Osteoarthritis is more common as people age.

Genetics: Some types of arthritis have a genetic component.

Injury: Joint injuries or trauma can increase the risk of developing arthritis.

Obesity: Excess weight puts additional stress on the joints, increasing the risk of osteoarthritis.

Autoimmune Disorders: Conditions like rheumatoid arthritis are autoimmune diseases where the immune system attacks the joints.

Treatment:

Treatment for arthritis depends on the type and severity of the condition. Common approaches include:

Medications: These may include pain relievers, anti-inflammatory drugs, and disease-modifying antirheumatic drugs (DMARDs) for inflammatory types of arthritis.

Physical Therapy: Exercises and physical therapy can help improve joint function and reduce pain.

Lifestyle Changes: Maintaining a healthy weight, eating an anti-inflammatory diet, and managing stress can help.

Surgery: In severe cases, joint replacement surgery may be necessary.

It's important for individuals with arthritis to work closely with healthcare professionals to develop a personalized treatment plan that addresses their specific needs and aims to improve their quality of life while managing the condition's symptoms. Early diagnosis and appropriate management can help individuals with arthritis lead active and fulfilling lives.

# Types of Arthritis

There are more than 100 different types of arthritis, each with its own characteristics, causes, and treatments. However, the two most common types of arthritis are osteoarthritis and rheumatoid arthritis. Here's an overview of these two prevalent types, along with a mention of a few other notable forms of arthritis:

Osteoarthritis (OA):

Description: Osteoarthritis is the most common form of arthritis and is often referred to as "wear and tear" arthritis. It primarily affects the joints where the protective cartilage that cushions the ends of bones wears down over time, leading to pain, swelling, and reduced joint flexibility.

Causes: Aging, joint injuries, obesity, and genetics are common risk factors. Overuse of joints due to repetitive motion or sports-related activities can also contribute.

Symptoms: Joint pain, stiffness (particularly in the morning or after periods of inactivity), reduced range of motion, and joint crepitus (cracking or grating sounds).

Treatment: Pain relief medication, physical therapy, lifestyle modifications (weight management and exercise), and in some cases, joint replacement surgery.

Rheumatoid Arthritis (RA):

Description: Rheumatoid arthritis is an autoimmune disorder in which the immune system mistakenly attacks the synovium, the lining of the membranes that surround the joints. This leads to inflammation, joint damage, and pain.

Causes: The exact cause is unknown, but genetics and environmental factors are believed to play a role.

Symptoms: Joint pain, swelling, stiffness, fatigue, and, over time, joint deformities.

Treatment: Disease-modifying antirheumatic drugs (DMARDs), nonsteroidal anti-inflammatory drugs (NSAIDs), physical therapy, and lifestyle changes are often used to manage RA.

Psoriatic Arthritis:

Description: Psoriatic arthritis is an autoimmune disease that affects some individuals with psoriasis, a skin condition characterized by red, scaly patches. It causes joint inflammation, pain, and can affect both the skin and joints.

Symptoms: Joint pain, skin lesions (psoriasis), swelling of fingers and toes, and nail changes.

Treatment: Medications to manage symptoms and slow the progression of the disease, physical therapy, and lifestyle modifications.

Ankylosing Spondylitis:

Description: Ankylosing spondylitis primarily affects the spine and sacroiliac joints, causing inflammation and stiffness. It often leads to a gradual fusion of the spine, limiting mobility.

Symptoms: Lower back pain, stiffness, and limited spinal mobility. It can also affect other joints and organs.

Treatment: Medications, physical therapy, and exercise to maintain flexibility.

Gout:

Description: Gout is characterized by the accumulation of urate crystals in the joints, leading to sudden and severe attacks of pain, redness, and swelling, typically in the big toe.

Causes: High levels of uric acid in the blood, often due to dietary choices.

Treatment: Medications to lower uric acid levels, lifestyle changes, and anti-inflammatory drugs to manage pain during attacks.

These are just a few examples of the many types of arthritis. Each type has its unique characteristics and may require different approaches to treatment and management. It's important for individuals with arthritis to work closely with healthcare professionals to receive a proper diagnosis and develop a personalized treatment plan

# Arthritis Symptoms and Diagnosis

Arthritis encompasses a wide range of conditions, and the symptoms can vary depending on the type of arthritis. However, there are some common symptoms that people with arthritis may experience. Here are the typical symptoms and the diagnostic process for arthritis:

Common Arthritis Symptoms:

Joint Pain: Persistent pain in one or more joints is a hallmark symptom of arthritis. The pain may be mild to severe and can be constant or intermittent.

Joint Swelling: Arthritis often leads to inflammation, resulting in swelling in the affected joints. Swelling can cause joint stiffness and discomfort.

Joint Stiffness: Many individuals with arthritis experience joint stiffness, especially in the morning or after periods of inactivity. This stiffness can make it difficult to move the affected joints.

Reduced Range of Motion: Arthritis can limit the range of motion in affected joints, making it challenging to perform everyday activities and affecting one's overall mobility.

Warmth and Redness: Inflamed joints may feel warm to the touch and appear red or flushed due to increased blood flow to the area.

Fatigue: Chronic pain and inflammation associated with arthritis can lead to fatigue, affecting a person's energy levels and daily activities.

Joint Deformities: Over time, untreated or poorly managed arthritis can lead to joint deformities, especially in conditions like rheumatoid arthritis.

Fever and Weight Loss: Some forms of inflammatory arthritis, like rheumatoid arthritis, may be accompanied by systemic symptoms, including fever and unexplained weight loss.

Diagnosis of Arthritis:

Medical History: The diagnostic process typically begins with a thorough medical history. Your healthcare provider will ask about your symptoms, their duration, and any family history of arthritis or related conditions.

Physical Examination: A physical examination is often conducted to assess joint tenderness, swelling, warmth, and range of motion. This can help identify areas of concern.

Blood Tests: Blood tests, such as the erythrocyte sedimentation rate (ESR) and C-reactive protein (CRP) tests, can help detect signs of inflammation in the body. Other tests may be used to check for specific antibodies in the case of autoimmune forms of arthritis.

Imaging: X-rays, MRI (Magnetic Resonance Imaging), or ultrasound may be used to visualize the affected joints and assess for joint damage or changes in the bone and soft tissues.

Synovial Fluid Analysis: In some cases, a sample of synovial fluid (the fluid that lubricates joints) may be aspirated and analyzed for signs of infection or inflammation.

Specialized Tests: For certain types of arthritis, specialized tests may be necessary. For example, the HLA-B27 test is used to diagnose ankylosing spondylitis.

It's important to note that there is no single definitive test for all types of arthritis, and diagnosis often involves a combination of clinical evaluation, lab tests, and imaging studies. Once diagnosed, healthcare providers can work with patients to develop a tailored treatment plan to manage the condition and improve the quality of life. Early diagnosis and treatment can be essential in preventing further joint damage and complications.

# Managing Arthritis Through Diet

Managing arthritis through diet is an essential aspect of overall arthritis care. While diet alone may not cure arthritis, it can play a significant role in reducing inflammation, managing symptoms, and improving the quality of life for individuals with arthritis. Here are some dietary strategies for managing arthritis:

Anti-Inflammatory Foods:

Include foods with anti-inflammatory properties in your diet. These foods can help reduce inflammation and alleviate arthritis symptoms. Examples include fatty fish (such as salmon, mackerel, and sardines), leafy greens (like spinach and kale), nuts, seeds, berries, and turmeric.

Omega-3 Fatty Acids:

Omega-3 fatty acids, found in fish, flaxseeds, and walnuts, have anti-inflammatory properties. Incorporate these sources into your diet regularly.

Healthy Fats:

Replace saturated and trans fats with healthier fats like those found in olive oil, avocados, and nuts. These fats can help reduce inflammation.

Fiber-Rich Foods:

Whole grains, fruits, and vegetables are rich in fiber, which can help maintain a healthy weight and reduce inflammation. Aim for a diet rich in fiber from these sources.

Colorful Fruits and Vegetables:

Choose a variety of colorful fruits and vegetables. They are packed with antioxidants and vitamins that can help combat inflammation and support overall health.

Lean Proteins:

Opt for lean sources of protein, such as skinless poultry, beans, lentils, and tofu. Limit your consumption of red meat, particularly processed meats.

Spices and Herbs:

Incorporate anti-inflammatory spices and herbs like ginger, garlic, cinnamon, and turmeric into your cooking. They can add flavor and health benefits to your meals.

Dairy Alternatives:

If you have lactose intolerance or dairy triggers your symptoms, consider dairy alternatives like almond milk or soy yogurt.

Hydration:

Stay well-hydrated by drinking plenty of water. Proper hydration helps maintain joint health and overall bodily functions.

Limit Sugar and Processed Foods:

Excess sugar and processed foods can contribute to inflammation. Reduce your consumption of sugary snacks, sugary drinks, and heavily processed foods.

Maintain a Healthy Weight:

Excess body weight can put added stress on joints, especially in weight-bearing joints like the knees and hips. Maintaining a healthy weight can reduce joint pain and improve mobility.

Consider Dietary Supplements:

Consult with a healthcare professional before taking dietary supplements. Some people with arthritis may benefit from supplements like glucosamine, chondroitin, or fish oil. However, individual needs vary.

Consult a Dietitian:

If you have specific dietary concerns or require personalized guidance, consider consulting a registered dietitian who specializes in arthritis and inflammatory conditions. They can help create a tailored nutrition plan.

It's essential to remember that dietary changes may take time to show results, and individual responses to certain foods can vary. Additionally, while diet can be a valuable part of arthritis management, it should be combined with other treatment strategies, including medication, physical therapy, and lifestyle modifications, as recommended by your healthcare provider.

# Chapter 1: Arthritis-Friendly Ingredients

# Anti-Inflammatory Foods

Anti-Inflammatory Foods: Your Path to Health and Wellness

Inflammation is a natural process that occurs in the body as a response to injury or infection. However, when inflammation becomes chronic and persists for extended periods, it can lead to various health issues, including heart disease, diabetes, and, notably, arthritis. Fortunately, one of the most effective ways to combat chronic inflammation is through your diet. Incorporating anti-inflammatory foods into your meals can play a significant role in managing conditions like arthritis and promoting overall health.

Understanding Inflammation: Acute vs. Chronic

Before we dive into the world of anti-inflammatory foods, it's essential to distinguish between acute and chronic inflammation:

Acute Inflammation: This type of inflammation is the body's immediate response to injury or infection. It serves as a protective mechanism, helping the body heal. Symptoms include redness, heat, swelling, and pain, which are all signs of increased blood flow to the affected area.

Chronic Inflammation: In contrast, chronic inflammation is a prolonged, low-level inflammatory response that can persist for months or even years. Unlike acute inflammation, it's not a helpful response and can harm the body's tissues. Chronic inflammation is often associated with various health conditions, including arthritis.

The Role of Diet in Inflammation

Diet plays a significant role in modulating inflammation. Certain foods can either promote or reduce inflammation within the body. The key lies in making choices that minimize the consumption of pro-inflammatory foods and maximize the intake of anti-inflammatory ones.

Anti-Inflammatory Foods: What to Include in Your Diet

Fatty Fish: Fish like salmon, mackerel, and sardines are rich in omega-3 fatty acids. These fats have powerful anti-inflammatory properties and can help reduce inflammation throughout the body.

Berries: Blueberries, strawberries, and raspberries are packed with antioxidants called flavonoids, which have been shown to combat inflammation.

Leafy Greens: Spinach, kale, and Swiss chard are excellent sources of antioxidants, vitamins, and minerals that can help reduce inflammation.

Nuts and Seeds: Almonds, walnuts, and flaxseeds contain healthy fats and antioxidants that combat inflammation.

Turmeric: Curcumin, the active compound in turmeric, is a potent anti-inflammatory agent. It's often used in curries and can be taken as a supplement.

Olive Oil: Extra virgin olive oil contains oleocanthal, which has similar anti-inflammatory properties to ibuprofen.

Whole Grains: Foods like brown rice, quinoa, and whole wheat bread are rich in fiber and can help reduce markers of inflammation.

Spices: Ginger, garlic, and cinnamon have anti-inflammatory properties and can be used to season your dishes.

Fruits: Cherries, oranges, and apples contain antioxidants and other compounds that can reduce inflammation.

Green Tea: The catechins in green tea have anti-inflammatory effects and can be a healthy beverage choice.

Foods to Limit or Avoid

In addition to incorporating anti-inflammatory foods, it's crucial to minimize or avoid foods that can promote inflammation. These include:

Processed Foods: Highly processed foods often contain trans fats, sugar, and artificial additives, all of which can contribute to inflammation.

Sugary Beverages: Soda, energy drinks, and excessive fruit juices can lead to inflammation due to their high sugar content.

Saturated and Trans Fats: Foods high in these fats, such as fried foods, processed meats, and certain dairy products, can promote inflammation.

Excessive Red Meat: While lean sources of red meat are acceptable in moderation, excessive consumption can lead to inflammation.

Conclusion

Incorporating a variety of anti-inflammatory foods into your diet is a proactive step toward managing chronic inflammation, such as that associated with arthritis. By making thoughtful choices and emphasizing whole, unprocessed foods, you can help reduce inflammation in your body and support your overall health and wellness. Remember that a balanced diet, in conjunction with any prescribed medical treatments, can be a powerful tool in your journey to managing arthritis and promoting long-term well-being.

# Omega-3 Fatty Acids

Omega-3 fatty acids are a type of polyunsaturated fat that is essential for good health. They are considered "essential" because the human body cannot produce them on its own; they must be obtained through diet. Omega-3 fatty acids play a crucial role in various bodily functions and have been associated with numerous health benefits, including heart health, brain function, and reducing inflammation. Let's explore omega-3 fatty acids in detail:

Types of Omega-3 Fatty Acids:

There are three main types of omega-3 fatty acids:

Alpha-Linolenic Acid (ALA): ALA is found in plant-based sources, such as flaxseeds, chia seeds, walnuts, and hemp seeds. It is considered the precursor to the other two types of omega-3s and must be converted by the body into eicosatetraenoic acid (EPA) and docosahexaenoic acid (DHA) to be fully utilized.

Eicosatetraenoic Acid (EPA): EPA is primarily found in fatty fish, such as salmon, mackerel, and sardines. It is known for its anti-inflammatory properties and is often recommended for cardiovascular health.

Docosahexaenoic Acid (DHA): DHA is also abundant in fatty fish and is particularly important for brain health and development. It plays a crucial role in maintaining the structure and function of brain cells.

Health Benefits of Omega-3 Fatty Acids:

Omega-3 fatty acids offer a wide range of health benefits:

Heart Health: Omega-3s are known to reduce the risk of heart disease. They can lower triglycerides, reduce blood pressure, decrease inflammation in blood vessels, and improve overall heart function.

Brain Function: DHA, in particular, is critical for brain health. It is a major component of brain cell membranes and is essential for cognitive function, memory, and concentration.

Mood and Mental Health: Some studies suggest that omega-3s may help reduce symptoms of depression, anxiety, and other mood disorders. They are thought to have a positive impact on neurotransmitter function in the brain.

Inflammation: Omega-3s have anti-inflammatory properties, making them valuable in managing inflammatory conditions such as arthritis. They can help reduce joint pain and stiffness.

Eye Health: DHA is present in high concentrations in the retina of the eye and is important for maintaining vision and preventing age-related eye diseases.

Pregnancy and Infant Development: Omega-3s, especially DHA, are critical during pregnancy for fetal brain and eye development. They are often included in prenatal supplements.

Sources of Omega-3 Fatty Acids:

To incorporate more omega-3 fatty acids into your diet, consider these sources:

Fatty Fish: Salmon, mackerel, sardines, trout, and herring are rich in EPA and DHA.

Plant-Based Sources: Flaxseeds, chia seeds, walnuts, hemp seeds, and algae-based supplements are high in ALA.

Fish Oil Supplements: Fish oil capsules or liquid supplements are available and can provide a concentrated source of EPA and DHA.

Recommended Dietary Intake:

The American Heart Association recommends eating two servings of fatty fish per week to obtain sufficient omega-3 fatty acids for heart health. For those who don't consume fish regularly, omega-3 supplements can be considered, but it's important to consult a healthcare professional before starting any supplementation regimen.

Conclusion:

Omega-3 fatty acids are vital for overall health, with numerous benefits for heart health, brain function, and reducing inflammation. Incorporating a variety of omega-3-rich foods into your diet can contribute to improved well-being. However, it's essential to maintain a balanced diet and consult with a healthcare provider before making significant dietary changes or starting supplements, especially if you have specific health concerns

# Foods to Limit or Avoid

To manage conditions like arthritis and promote overall health, it's essential to be mindful of foods that may exacerbate inflammation and negatively impact your well-being. Here are types of foods to limit or avoid in your diet:

1. Processed Foods:

Why to Limit: Processed foods often contain high levels of refined sugars, unhealthy fats, artificial additives, and preservatives, all of which can contribute to inflammation and overall poor health.

Examples: Sugary cereals, sugary snacks, pre-packaged frozen meals, and fast food.

2. Sugary Beverages:

Why to Limit: Sugar-sweetened beverages, including soda, energy drinks, and certain fruit juices, are loaded with added sugars that can promote inflammation, contribute to weight gain, and increase the risk of chronic diseases.

Alternatives: Choose water, herbal tea, or unsweetened beverages to stay hydrated.

3. Saturated and Trans Fats:

Why to Limit: Saturated fats, found in red meat, full-fat dairy products, and processed foods, can promote inflammation and raise cholesterol levels. Trans fats, often found in partially hydrogenated oils, have been linked to various health problems, including heart disease.

Alternatives: Opt for lean cuts of meat, low-fat dairy, and foods prepared with healthier fats like olive oil.

4. Red and Processed Meats:

Why to Limit: Red and processed meats can contain saturated fats and advanced glycation end products (AGEs), which can promote inflammation and oxidative stress.

Alternatives: Choose lean protein sources like poultry, fish, legumes, and plant-based protein options.

5. Refined Carbohydrates:

Why to Limit: Refined carbohydrates, such as white bread, white rice, and sugary cereals, have a high glycemic index and can lead to rapid spikes in blood sugar levels, potentially worsening inflammation.

Alternatives: Opt for whole grains like brown rice, quinoa, and whole wheat bread.

6. Excessive Alcohol:

Why to Limit: Excessive alcohol consumption can contribute to inflammation and negatively affect the immune system. It can also interact with certain medications used to manage arthritis.

Moderation: If you choose to consume alcohol, do so in moderation and be mindful of potential interactions with medications.

7. Foods High in Salt (Sodium):

Why to Limit: High-sodium foods can lead to water retention and may exacerbate joint swelling and inflammation.

Alternatives: Use herbs and spices for flavoring instead of salt, and choose low-sodium or salt-free versions of canned and packaged foods.

8. Artificial Trans Fats:

Why to Avoid: Artificial trans fats, often found in some margarines and baked goods, have been banned or restricted in many countries due to their negative health impact, including inflammation and heart disease.

9. Nightshade Vegetables (for Some Individuals):


Why to Limit (for Some): Some individuals with certain types of arthritis, like rheumatoid arthritis, report symptom improvement when they limit or avoid nightshade vegetables, including tomatoes, potatoes, peppers, and eggplants. However, this varies from person to person, and more research is needed in this area.

10. Dairy Products (for Some Individuals):

- Why to Limit (for Some): Dairy products can trigger symptoms in some individuals with arthritis. If you suspect dairy worsens your symptoms, you may consider dairy alternatives like almond milk or lactose-free products.


Conclusion:

While these foods are best limited or avoided to help manage inflammation and promote overall health, it's essential to work with a healthcare provider or a registered dietitian to create a personalized dietary plan that aligns with your specific health needs and any existing medical conditions, including arthritis. A balanced and nutritious diet tailored to your unique requirements can be a valuable part of your arthritis management strategy.

# Chapter 2: Kitchen Essentials for Arthritis Patients

## Ergonomic Kitchen Tools

Ergonomic kitchen tools are designed to make cooking tasks more comfortable, efficient, and safe while reducing the risk of strain or injury. These tools are especially valuable for individuals with arthritis or other conditions that affect hand and wrist mobility. Here's a detailed overview of ergonomic kitchen tools and their benefits:

1. Ergonomic Utensils:

Description: Ergonomic utensils have specially designed handles that are comfortable to grip and reduce strain on the hand and wrist. They often have a contoured shape and non-slip surfaces.

Benefits: These utensils make it easier to hold and control while stirring, flipping, or serving food. They can be particularly helpful for individuals with arthritis or hand weakness.

2. Ergonomic Knives:

Description: Ergonomic knives feature handles with an ergonomic shape that promotes a natural wrist position. Some have textured grips for better control.

Benefits: They reduce the strain on the wrist and hand when cutting, chopping, or slicing, making these tasks more comfortable and safer. They are particularly useful for individuals with arthritis or carpal tunnel syndrome.

3. Ergonomic Can Openers:

Description: Ergonomic can openers have large, comfortable handles and a design that minimizes the effort required to open cans.

Benefits: They are easier to grip and turn, making it more accessible for individuals with hand pain or weakness. Some models also have a magnetic lid lifter for added convenience.

4. Ergonomic Peeler:

Description: Ergonomic peelers are designed with a comfortable handle and a swivel blade that follows the contours of fruits and vegetables.

Benefits: They reduce hand and wrist strain when peeling, and their design minimizes the need to apply excessive pressure. This is especially helpful for those with arthritis or repetitive strain injuries.

5. Ergonomic Cutting Boards:

Description: These cutting boards often have non-slip bases and may come with a raised or tilted design to make chopping and slicing easier.

Benefits: They provide stability, reduce the need for excessive force, and maintain a more comfortable hand and wrist position while cutting. Some also have built-in knife guides for added safety.

6. Ergonomic Graters:

Description: Ergonomic graters have handles designed for a more comfortable grip and may include rubberized bases for stability during grating.

Benefits: They reduce hand fatigue and make grating tasks less strenuous. The stable base ensures that the grater remains steady during use.

7. Ergonomic Jar and Bottle Openers:

Description: These tools are designed to grip and open jars, bottles, and containers with minimal effort. They often have rubberized or contoured handles.

Benefits: They provide extra leverage and grip, making it easier to twist and open tightly sealed containers. This is particularly useful for individuals with hand or wrist issues.

8. Ergonomic Mixing Bowls:

Description: Ergonomic mixing bowls come with non-slip bases and easy-grip handles to facilitate mixing, pouring, and holding.

Benefits: They enhance stability and control during food preparation, reducing the risk of spills and making tasks like stirring and pouring more manageable.

9. Ergonomic Kitchen Gadgets:

Description: Various kitchen gadgets, such as garlic presses, can openers, and egg slicers, come in ergonomic designs with user-friendly handles.

Benefits: These gadgets are more comfortable to hold and use, making specific tasks less strenuous and more accessible for individuals with hand or wrist discomfort.

Conclusion:

Ergonomic kitchen tools are valuable aids for improving comfort and safety in the kitchen, especially for individuals with arthritis or hand-related challenges. When choosing ergonomic tools, consider your specific needs and preferences to create a kitchen environment that is both functional and accommodating.

# Meal Preparation Tips

Meal preparation, also known as meal prep, is the process of planning and preparing meals in advance. It's a practical and time-saving approach that can help you eat healthier, save money, and reduce stress during the week. Here are detailed meal preparation tips to help you get started:

1. Set Clear Goals:

Determine why you want to meal prep. It could be to save time, eat healthier, or stick to a specific dietary plan. Having clear goals will guide your meal prep efforts.

2. Plan Your Meals:

Create a meal plan for the week. Decide which meals you want to prepare in advance, such as breakfast, lunch, dinner, and snacks. Consider your dietary preferences, nutritional needs, and any dietary restrictions.

3. Choose Balanced Recipes:

Select recipes that provide a balance of protein, carbohydrates, healthy fats, and a variety of vegetables. This ensures that your meals are nutritious and satisfying.

4. Make a Shopping List:

Based on your meal plan, create a shopping list of all the ingredients you'll need. Organize the list by categories to make grocery shopping efficient.

5. Invest in Quality Containers:

Use a variety of food storage containers that are microwave-safe, dishwasher-safe, and airtight. Having the right containers makes it easier to portion and store your meals.

6. Cook in Batches:

Prepare larger quantities of key components like grains, proteins, and vegetables. Cook once and use these ingredients in multiple meals throughout the week.

7. Use Time-Saving Appliances:

Utilize kitchen appliances like slow cookers, instant pots, and air fryers to streamline cooking processes. These appliances can save time and make meal prep more convenient.

8. Prep Vegetables in Advance:

Wash, chop, and store vegetables in portion-sized containers. Having prepped veggies on hand makes it quick and easy to add them to meals.

9. Portion Control:

Use a kitchen scale or measuring cups to ensure accurate portion sizes. This helps with calorie control and prevents overeating.

10. Cook Proteins Thoroughly:

- When preparing proteins (e.g., chicken, fish, or beans), ensure they are cooked thoroughly to prevent foodborne illnesses. Invest in a food thermometer to check internal temperatures.

11. Label and Date Meals:

- Label containers with the meal's name and date of preparation. This helps you keep track of freshness and ensures you use older meals first.

12. Freeze Meals for Later:

- If you're preparing meals for the entire week, consider freezing some portions to maintain freshness. Make sure to use freezer-safe containers.

13. Rotate Ingredients:

- To prevent food waste, try to incorporate ingredients from your pantry and refrigerator into your meal prep. Use items that are close to their expiration date.

14. Stay Organized:

- Keep your kitchen organized and clean while meal prepping. This will help you work efficiently and minimize stress.

15. Schedule Meal Prep Time:

- Dedicate a specific time each week for meal prep. Consistency will make it easier to incorporate into your routine.

16. Be Creative:

- Don't be afraid to experiment with different recipes and cuisines. Variety can make meal prep more enjoyable and prevent boredom with your meals.

### 17. Plan for Snacks:

- Prepare healthy snacks like cut-up fruit, yogurt, or nuts to avoid reaching for less nutritious options when you're hungry between meals.

### 18. Practice Food Safety:

- Maintain proper food safety practices, such as washing hands, sanitizing surfaces, and refrigerating perishable items promptly.

### 19. Enjoy Your Meals:

- Take the time to savor your prepared meals. Meal prep should enhance your eating experience, not just save time.

### 20. Evaluate and Adjust:

- Periodically review your meal prep process. Adjust your meal plan, recipes, or strategies based on what works best for you and your goals.

Meal preparation is a valuable skill that can improve your eating habits, save you time, and reduce food waste. With careful planning and practice, you can make meal prep an enjoyable and sustainable part of your routine.

# Storage and Organization

Effective storage and organization in the kitchen are essential for keeping your cooking space functional, efficient, and clutter-free. Whether you have a small kitchen or a spacious one, good organization can make meal prep and cooking much more enjoyable. Here are detailed tips for storage and organization in the kitchen:

1. Declutter Your Kitchen:

Start by going through your kitchen and decluttering items you no longer use or need. This includes expired food, broken appliances, and kitchen tools you rarely use. Donate or discard what you don't need.

2. Maximize Cabinet Space:

Utilize adjustable shelves in cabinets to accommodate various-sized items. Consider installing pull-out shelves or drawers for easier access to pots, pans, and other cookware.

3. Organize Pantry Items:

Categorize and label pantry items. Store frequently used items at eye level and less frequently used items on higher or lower shelves. Use clear containers for grains, pasta, and dry goods to keep them visible and prevent pantry pests.

4. Use Drawer Dividers:

Drawer dividers or inserts are great for keeping utensils, cutlery, and kitchen gadgets organized. They prevent items from getting mixed up and make it easy to find what you need.

5. Invest in Shelving Units:

If you have limited cabinet space, consider adding open shelving units on walls. These can hold dishes, glassware, and decorative kitchen items, adding both storage and style to your kitchen.

6. Store Items by Function:

Group kitchen items by function and store them accordingly. For example, keep baking supplies like flour, sugar, and baking sheets in one area, and cooking utensils, pots, and pans in another.

7. Use Clear Containers:

Store leftovers, bulk ingredients, or snacks in clear, airtight containers. This makes it easy to see the contents and helps keep food fresh longer.

8. Hang Pots and Pans:

Hang pots, pans, and kitchen utensils on a wall-mounted rack or hooks to free up cabinet space and keep them within easy reach.

9. Install a Pegboard:

Pegboards are versatile and can be customized with hooks and shelves to store a variety of kitchen items, from pots and pans to cutting boards and utensils.

10. Store Knives Safely:

- Use a knife block or magnetic strip to store knives safely and keep them organized and accessible.

11. Utilize Lazy Susans:

- Lazy Susans are excellent for corner cabinets or deep pantry shelves. They allow you to access items easily without reaching to the back of the shelf.

12. Create Zones:

- Organize your kitchen into zones based on function, such as a baking zone, cooking zone, and cleaning zone. Keep related items and tools together for efficiency.

13. Label Everything:

- Label containers, drawers, and shelves to ensure that everything has a designated place. Labels make it easier to find what you need and maintain organization.

14. Stack Vertically:

- Opt for stackable containers and nesting bowls and pots to save space and keep your kitchen neat.

15. Utilize Door Space:

- Attach organizers to the inside of cabinet doors for storing spices, lids, or cleaning supplies.

16. Use Under-Cabinet Lighting:

- Installing under-cabinet lighting can improve visibility and make it easier to find items in dark or dimly lit areas of the kitchen.

17. Maintain Regular Cleaning:

- Regularly clean and declutter your kitchen to prevent clutter from building up. Wipe down surfaces and appliances, and empty the dishwasher and trash regularly.


18. Rotate Items:

- Periodically rotate pantry items and check for expiration dates. Use older items first to minimize food waste.


19. Seek Inspiration:

- Look for kitchen organization inspiration online or in-home improvement magazines to discover creative storage solutions and design ideas.


20. Personalize Your Kitchen:

- Organize your kitchen in a way that works best for you and your cooking habits. Customization ensures that everything is accessible and efficient.


Effective storage and organization in the kitchen can save you time, reduce stress, and make cooking and meal prep more enjoyable. Tailor your organization strategy to your kitchen's layout and your specific needs to create a well-organized and functional cooking space.

# Chapter 3: Breakfast Delights

## Berry Blast Smoothie

A Berry Blast Smoothie is a delightful and nutritious beverage that combines the goodness of various berries with other ingredients to create a refreshing and healthful drink. This smoothie is not only delicious but also packed with antioxidants, vitamins, and fiber. Here's a detailed recipe and guide on how to make a Berry Blast Smoothie:

Ingredients:

1. Mixed Berries: Use a combination of your favorite berries. Common choices include strawberries, blueberries, raspberries, and blackberries. You can use fresh or frozen berries.

2. Greek Yogurt: Greek yogurt adds creaminess, protein, and a tangy flavor to the smoothie. You can use plain or flavored yogurt, depending on your preference.

3. Banana: A ripe banana not only adds natural sweetness but also provides a creamy texture to the smoothie.

4. Liquid: You'll need a liquid to blend the ingredients smoothly. Options include milk (dairy or plant-based), yogurt, or fruit juice. Adjust the quantity to achieve your desired consistency.

5. Honey or Sweetener (Optional): Depending on your taste preference, you can add a touch of honey, agave syrup, or another sweetener if you want a sweeter smoothie.

6. Ice (Optional): If you prefer a colder and thicker smoothie, consider adding ice cubes.

Instructions:

1. Prepare Your Ingredients:

Wash the berries thoroughly if using fresh ones. If you're using frozen berries, there's no need to thaw them. Peel and slice the banana.

2. Combine Ingredients:

In a blender, add the mixed berries, sliced banana, and Greek yogurt.

3. Add Liquid:

Pour in your chosen liquid. The quantity depends on how thick or thin you want your smoothie to be. Start with a small amount and add more as needed.

4. Sweeten to Taste:

If you desire extra sweetness, add honey or your preferred sweetener at this stage.

5. Blend Until Smooth:

Start blending on low speed and gradually increase to high. Blend until all the ingredients are well combined and the smoothie is creamy and smooth.

6. Check Consistency:

If your smoothie is too thick, add more liquid and blend again. If it's too thin, you can add more frozen berries or ice cubes and blend until you achieve the desired consistency.

7. Serve and Enjoy:

Pour your Berry Blast Smoothie into a glass or a to-go cup. You can garnish it with a few fresh berries or a slice of banana if you like. Serve immediately while it's fresh and cold.

Tips:

Customize your Berry Blast Smoothie by adding extras like chia seeds, flax seeds, or spinach for added nutrition.

To make it even more refreshing, you can use frozen yogurt or ice cream instead of Greek yogurt.

Adjust the sweetness to your liking. You can also use natural sweeteners like maple syrup or stevia.

If you prefer a dairy-free option, use almond milk, soy milk, or coconut milk as the liquid base.

A Berry Blast Smoothie is a versatile and healthy choice for breakfast, a snack, or a post-workout refreshment. It's packed with vitamins, antioxidants, and natural sweetness from the berries and banana, making it both delicious and nutritious. Feel free to get creative with your Berry Blast Smoothie by experimenting with different berry combinations and toppings.

# Overnight Oats with Almonds

Overnight oats with almonds is a nutritious and convenient breakfast option that combines the creaminess of oats with the crunch and nutty flavor of almonds. This dish can be customized to suit your taste preferences and dietary needs, making it a versatile and satisfying breakfast. Here's a detailed guide on how to make overnight oats with almonds:

Ingredients:

1. Rolled Oats: Rolled oats are the base of this dish. They are whole-grain oats that have been flattened to make them cook faster and have a pleasant texture.

2. Almonds: Almonds add a delightful crunch and nutty flavor to the oats. You can use whole almonds or sliced almonds, and you have the option to toast them for extra flavor.

3. Milk: You can use your choice of milk, whether it's dairy milk, almond milk, soy milk, or any other plant-based milk. Use unsweetened milk for a healthier option.

4. Sweetener (Optional): If you like your oats sweeter, you can add a natural sweetener like honey, maple syrup, agave nectar, or stevia.

5. Yogurt (Optional): Greek yogurt or any yogurt of your choice can be added for creaminess and a touch of tanginess.

6. Fruits (Optional): Fresh or dried fruits like berries, sliced bananas, chopped apples, or raisins can be included for added flavor and nutrition.

7. Spices: You can add a pinch of cinnamon or a dash of vanilla extract for extra flavor.

Instructions:

1. Prepare the Almonds:

If you'd like to toast the almonds, place them in a dry skillet over medium heat. Stir frequently until they become fragrant and lightly browned. Remove them from the heat and let them cool before chopping or using them whole.

2. Combine Ingredients:

In a container or jar with a lid, combine the rolled oats, chopped or whole almonds, and any sweetener or spices you'd like to include.

3. Add Milk and Yogurt:

Pour in the milk of your choice. If you're using yogurt, add it to the mixture as well. The amount of liquid you use will depend on your desired oat-to-liquid ratio. A common ratio is 1:1, but you can adjust it to your liking.

4. Mix Well:

Stir the ingredients together until everything is well combined. Make sure the oats are fully submerged in the liquid.

5. Refrigerate Overnight:

Seal the container or jar with a lid and place it in the refrigerator. Let the oats and almonds soak and absorb the liquid overnight, or for at least 4-6 hours. This allows the oats to soften and become creamy.

6. Serve and Customize:

The next morning, or when you're ready to eat, give the oats a good stir. You can add fresh or dried fruits at this point for added flavor and texture.

7. Garnish with Almonds:

To enhance the almond flavor and provide an extra crunch, sprinkle additional almonds on top before serving.

8. Enjoy:

Your overnight oats with almonds are now ready to be enjoyed. Eat them cold straight from the refrigerator, or you can warm them in the microwave for a warm and comforting breakfast.

Tips:

Experiment with different types of nuts or seeds, such as walnuts, pecans, or chia seeds, to vary the texture and flavor.

Customize your overnight oats with your favorite fruits, such as sliced strawberries, blueberries, or diced mango.

Adjust the sweetness to your preference by adding more or less sweetener.

To make your oats even creamier, use a combination of yogurt and milk.

Store leftover overnight oats in the refrigerator for up to two days.

Overnight oats with almonds are a convenient and nutritious breakfast option that can be prepared in advance, making busy mornings more manageable. Feel free to get creative with your toppings and flavorings to create a personalized and satisfying breakfast experience.

# Spinach and Mushroom Omelette

A spinach and mushroom omelette is a delicious and nutritious breakfast option that combines the earthy flavors of mushrooms, the vibrant green goodness of spinach, and the creamy texture of eggs. It's a protein-packed meal that can be customized to suit your taste. Here's a detailed guide on how to make a spinach and mushroom omelette:

Ingredients:

For the Omelette:

1. Eggs: You'll need two to three large eggs per omelette, depending on your preference and hunger level.

2. Spinach: Fresh baby spinach leaves work well in this recipe. You can also use frozen spinach, but be sure to thaw and squeeze out excess moisture before use.

3. Mushrooms: Sliced button mushrooms or your choice of mushroom variety (e.g., cremini, shiitake) add a savory depth of flavor to the omelette.

4. Onion (Optional): Chopped onions can be added for extra flavor and sweetness.

5. Garlic (Optional): Minced garlic cloves can enhance the overall taste of the omelette.

6. Butter or Oil: Use butter or a cooking oil of your choice (e.g., olive oil) to sauté the vegetables and prevent sticking.

7. Salt and Pepper: Season the omelette to taste with salt and freshly ground black pepper.

For Filling and Garnish (Optional):

8. Cheese: Grated cheese (e.g., cheddar, Swiss, feta) can be added for creaminess and flavor.

9. Herbs: Fresh herbs like parsley, chives, or basil can be sprinkled on top for a burst of freshness.

Instructions:

1. Prepare the Vegetables:

If using fresh spinach, wash and chop it. Slice the mushrooms, chop the onion (if using), and mince the garlic (if using).

2. Sauté the Vegetables:

In a non-stick skillet over medium heat, add a small amount of butter or oil. Add the chopped onion (if using) and sauté until it becomes translucent. Then, add the sliced mushrooms and minced garlic (if using) and cook until the mushrooms release their moisture and become tender.

Add the chopped spinach to the skillet and sauté for another minute or until it wilts. Season with salt and pepper to taste. Remove the vegetables from the skillet and set them aside.

3. Beat the Eggs:

In a bowl, beat the eggs until the yolks and whites are well combined. Season the eggs with a pinch of salt and pepper.

4. Cook the Omelette:

Wipe the skillet clean and return it to medium-low heat. Add a small amount of butter or oil to coat the bottom of the skillet.

Pour the beaten eggs into the skillet and let them cook undisturbed for a minute or until they start to set around the edges.

5. Add the Fillings:

Once the edges of the eggs begin to set, add the sautéed mushroom, spinach, and any cheese you'd like in the center of the omelette.

6. Fold the Omelette:

Gently lift one side of the omelette with a spatula and fold it over the fillings to create a half-moon shape.

7. Finish Cooking:

Continue cooking for another minute or until the omelette is fully set but still slightly runny on top. You can cover the skillet with a lid to help the top cook evenly.

8. Serve and Garnish:

Carefully slide the omelette onto a plate. Garnish with fresh herbs if desired.

9. Enjoy:

Your spinach and mushroom omelette is ready to be enjoyed. Serve it hot with toast, a side of fresh fruit, or your favorite breakfast accompaniments.

Tips:

Customize your omelette with other ingredients like diced bell peppers, diced tomatoes, or chopped ham.

Be cautious when adding salt, as the cheese and other ingredients may already add saltiness to the omelette.

If you prefer a fluffy omelette, you can separate the egg whites from the yolks, beat the whites until they form stiff peaks, and then fold in the yolks before cooking.

Experiment with different cheese varieties to vary the flavor and creaminess of your omelette.

For a dairy-free version, skip the cheese and use olive oil or dairy-free butter.

A spinach and mushroom omelette is a wholesome and satisfying breakfast option that's packed with protein and essential nutrients. It's a versatile dish that can be tailored to your taste, making it a delightful morning meal.

# Chapter 4: Soups and Salads

## Butternut Squash Soup

Butternut squash soup is a comforting and hearty dish that's perfect for cooler days. This creamy and flavorful soup combines the natural sweetness of roasted butternut squash with aromatic spices and other ingredients for a satisfying bowl of goodness. Here's a detailed guide on how to make butternut squash soup:

Ingredients:

1. Butternut Squash: You'll need one medium-sized butternut squash, which is approximately 2-3 pounds. You can also use pre-cut butternut squash to save time.

2. Onion: One medium onion, finely chopped, adds flavor and depth to the soup.

3. Garlic: Two to three cloves of garlic, minced, for a savory aroma.

4. Vegetable or Chicken Broth: Use around 4 cups of vegetable or chicken broth for the base of the soup. You can adjust the amount to achieve your desired consistency.

5. Olive Oil: For roasting the squash and sautéing the onions and garlic.

6. Spices: Common spices include ground cinnamon, nutmeg, and a pinch of cayenne pepper for a subtle kick. Salt and black pepper to taste.

7. Heavy Cream (Optional): To add richness and creaminess to the soup, you can include ½ cup of heavy cream. For a lighter version, substitute with coconut milk or omit the cream altogether.

8. Fresh Herbs (Optional): Chopped fresh herbs like thyme, rosemary, or sage can be used as a garnish for added flavor.

Instructions:

1. Prepare the Squash:

Preheat your oven to 400°F (200°C). Cut the butternut squash in half lengthwise and scoop out the seeds and fibers. You can save the seeds for roasting as a garnish if desired.

2. Roast the Squash:

Place the squash halves, cut-side up, on a baking sheet. Drizzle with olive oil, season with salt, pepper, and a pinch of cinnamon and nutmeg. Roast in the oven for about 45-60 minutes or until the squash is fork-tender and caramelized around the edges.

3. Sauté Onions and Garlic:

While the squash is roasting, heat some olive oil in a large soup pot over medium heat. Add the chopped onions and sauté until they become translucent, about 5-7 minutes. Add the minced garlic and continue to cook for another minute or until fragrant.

4. Scoop Out the Squash:

Once the squash is done roasting, let it cool slightly, and then scoop the flesh out of the skin. Transfer the roasted squash to the soup pot with the sautéed onions and garlic.

5. Blend the Soup:

Add the vegetable or chicken broth to the pot and bring the mixture to a simmer. Let it cook for about 10-15 minutes to meld the flavors.

Using an immersion blender or a regular blender, carefully puree the soup until smooth. If using a regular blender, do it in batches and be cautious with hot liquids. You can also use a potato masher for a chunkier texture.

6. Add Cream (Optional):

If you want to add creaminess, stir in the heavy cream or coconut milk at this stage. Simmer for an additional 5 minutes.

7. Season and Serve:

Season the soup with salt, pepper, and a pinch of cayenne pepper for a hint of heat. Adjust the seasoning to taste.

Serve the butternut squash soup hot, garnished with fresh herbs and a drizzle of cream if desired.

Tips:

To save time, you can use pre-cut butternut squash or even frozen butternut squash cubes.

Customize your soup with additional spices like ground ginger, allspice, or curry powder for different flavor profiles.

For a vegan version, use vegetable broth and coconut milk instead of cream.

Serve the soup with a dollop of Greek yogurt, croutons, or a sprinkle of grated Parmesan cheese for added texture and flavor.

Store leftover soup in an airtight container in the refrigerator for up to 3-4 days or freeze it for longer storage.

Butternut squash soup is a comforting and versatile dish that can be enjoyed as a starter or a satisfying meal. Its natural sweetness, combined with aromatic spices, makes it a delightful addition to your fall and winter menu.

# Quinoa and Kale Salad

A quinoa and kale salad are a nutritious and hearty dish that combines the protein-packed goodness of quinoa with the vibrant, leafy greens of kale. This salad is not only delicious but also versatile, as you can customize it with various toppings, dressings, and additional ingredients. Here's a detailed guide on how to make a quinoa and kale salad:

Ingredients:

For the Salad:

1. Quinoa: Use 1 cup of uncooked quinoa, which will yield approximately 3 cups of cooked quinoa. Rinse the quinoa thoroughly before cooking.

2. Kale: You'll need a bunch of fresh kale, preferably curly kale or lacinato kale (also known as dinosaur kale), with the tough stems removed and leaves chopped.

3. Vegetables: You can add a variety of colorful vegetables like bell peppers, cherry tomatoes, cucumber, or shredded carrots. Chop or slice them to your preferred size.

4. Nuts and Seeds: Toasted nuts (such as almonds, walnuts, or pecans) and seeds (like sunflower seeds or pumpkin seeds) add crunch and flavor to the salad.

5. Cheese (Optional): Crumbled feta, goat cheese, or grated Parmesan can provide a creamy and salty element to the salad.

For the Dressing:

6. Olive Oil: Use extra-virgin olive oil as the base for the dressing.

7. Lemon Juice: Freshly squeezed lemon juice adds a bright and tangy flavor to the dressing.

8. Dijon Mustard: A small amount of Dijon mustard emulsifies the dressing and enhances its flavor.

9. Honey (Optional): For sweetness, you can add a teaspoon of honey or maple syrup to balance the acidity.

10. Garlic: One clove of garlic, minced, for a subtle savory note.

11. Salt and Pepper: Season the dressing with salt and freshly ground black pepper to taste.

Instructions:

1. Cook Quinoa:

Rinse the quinoa under cold running water to remove any bitterness. In a saucepan, combine the rinsed quinoa and 2 cups of water. Bring to a boil, then reduce the heat to low, cover, and simmer for about 15-20 minutes, or until the quinoa is tender and the water is absorbed. Let it cool.

2. Massage Kale:

Place the chopped kale in a large mixing bowl. Drizzle with a small amount of olive oil and a pinch of salt. Massage the kale with your hands for a few minutes until it becomes tender and wilted. This step helps reduce the bitterness and improves the texture.

3. Prepare Vegetables, Nuts, and Seeds:

Chop or slice the vegetables and toast the nuts and seeds in a dry skillet over medium heat until they become fragrant and slightly browned. Let them cool.

4. Make Dressing:

In a small bowl, whisk together the olive oil, lemon juice, Dijon mustard, minced garlic, honey (if using), salt, and pepper. Adjust the seasoning to taste.

5. Assemble the Salad:

In a large salad bowl, combine the cooked quinoa, massaged kale, chopped vegetables, toasted nuts, and seeds. Toss everything together to distribute the ingredients evenly.

6. Add Cheese (Optional):

If you're using cheese, crumble or sprinkle it over the salad and gently toss.

7. Dress the Salad:

Pour the dressing over the salad and toss to coat all the ingredients with the dressing. Start with a small amount of dressing and add more as needed.

8. Serve and Enjoy:

Your quinoa and kale salad is ready to be served. It can be enjoyed immediately or refrigerated for a few hours to allow the flavors to meld. Serve it as a side dish or a main course.

Tips:

Customize your salad by adding protein sources like grilled chicken, chickpeas, or tofu for a more substantial meal.

Experiment with different herbs and spices in the dressing, such as fresh basil, oregano, or red pepper flakes, to vary the flavor profile.

To make this salad vegan, omit the cheese and use maple syrup instead of honey in the dressing.

Massage the kale just before serving to maintain its freshness and prevent it from becoming soggy.

Store leftover salad in an airtight container in the refrigerator for up to 2-3 days.

# Creamy Tomato Basil Soup

Creamy tomato basil soup is a classic and comforting dish that combines the rich, velvety texture of a tomato-based soup with the fresh, aromatic flavors of basil. This soup is perfect for a cozy meal, and it's easy to make from scratch. Here's a detailed guide on how to prepare creamy tomato basil soup:

Ingredients:

For the Soup:

1. Tomatoes: You can use either fresh tomatoes or canned tomatoes. If using fresh tomatoes, you'll need about 6-8 medium-sized tomatoes, chopped. If using canned tomatoes, opt for whole, peeled tomatoes.

2. Onion: One medium onion, finely chopped, adds sweetness and depth to the soup.

3. Garlic: Three to four cloves of garlic, minced, provide a rich, savory flavor.

4. Basil: Fresh basil leaves, chopped, add a vibrant herbal note to the soup. Reserve some leaves for garnish.

5. Vegetable or Chicken Broth: Use approximately 4 cups of vegetable or chicken broth as the base of the soup. You can adjust the amount to achieve your preferred consistency.

6. Heavy Cream (Optional): To add creaminess and richness to the soup, you can include ½ cup of heavy cream. For a lighter version, use half-and-half or omit the cream entirely.

7. Olive Oil: For sautéing the onions and garlic.

8. Salt and Pepper: Season the soup with salt and freshly ground black pepper to taste.

For the Garnish:

9. Fresh Basil Leaves: Reserved fresh basil leaves for garnish.

10. Croutons (Optional): Crispy croutons can be added for a delightful crunch.

11. Parmesan Cheese (Optional): Grated Parmesan cheese can be sprinkled on top for extra flavor.

Instructions:

1. Prepare the Tomatoes:

If using fresh tomatoes, wash and chop them. If using canned tomatoes, simply drain them and set aside.

2. Sauté Onions and Garlic:

In a large soup pot, heat some olive oil over medium heat. Add the chopped onion and sauté until it becomes translucent, about 5-7 minutes. Add the minced garlic and continue to cook for another minute until fragrant.

3. Add Tomatoes and Basil:

Add the chopped fresh tomatoes (or canned tomatoes) to the pot. If using fresh tomatoes, cook until they start to break down and release their juices, about 10-15 minutes. Stir in the chopped basil.

4. Blend the Soup:

Use an immersion blender or transfer the soup to a regular blender, working in batches if necessary. Blend until the soup is smooth and velvety.

5. Return to Heat:

Return the blended soup to the pot and place it over low to medium heat.

6. Add Broth:

Pour in the vegetable or chicken broth and stir to combine. Let the soup simmer for about 10-15 minutes to allow the flavors to meld.

7. Add Cream (Optional):

If you want to add creaminess, stir in the heavy cream or half-and-half at this stage. Simmer for an additional 5 minutes.

8. Season and Serve:

Season the soup with salt and freshly ground black pepper to taste. Adjust the seasoning as needed.

9. Garnish and Serve:

Ladle the creamy tomato basil soup into bowls. Garnish each serving with fresh basil leaves, croutons (if using), and grated Parmesan cheese (if desired).

10. Enjoy:

Your creamy tomato basil soup is ready to be enjoyed. Serve it hot with a slice of crusty bread for a comforting meal.

Tips:

Customize your soup by adding a pinch of red pepper flakes for a subtle heat or a drizzle of balsamic vinegar for extra depth of flavor.

For a vegan version, omit the cream and use olive oil instead of butter for sautéing the onions and garlic.

To make the soup smoother, you can strain it through a fine-mesh sieve after blending to remove any tomato skins or seeds.

Store leftover soup in an airtight container in the refrigerator for up to 3-4 days. Reheat it gently on the stovetop or in the microwave before serving.

Creamy tomato basil soup is a classic favorite that's simple to make and bursting with flavor. It's a perfect choice for a comforting lunch or dinner, especially when paired with your favorite bread or a grilled cheese sandwich.

# Chapter 5: Light and Satisfying Snacks

## Roasted Red Pepper Hummus

Roasted red pepper hummus is a flavorful and nutritious dip that combines the earthy taste of chickpeas with the smoky sweetness of roasted red peppers. This creamy and savory spread is perfect for dipping pita bread, fresh vegetables, or as a spread on sandwiches and wraps. Here's a detailed guide on how to make roasted red pepper hummus:

Ingredients:

For the Roasted Red Peppers:

1. Red Bell Peppers: You'll need 2 large red bell peppers to roast. You can also use jarred roasted red peppers to save time.

For the Hummus:

2. Chickpeas: One can (about 15 ounces) of chickpeas, drained and rinsed. You can also use cooked dried chickpeas.

3. Tahini: 1/4 cup of tahini (sesame paste) adds creaminess and nuttiness to the hummus.

4. Lemon Juice: Juice from 1 lemon (approximately 2-3 tablespoons) for tanginess.

5. Garlic: One or two cloves of garlic, minced, for a savory kick.

6. Olive Oil: 2-3 tablespoons of extra-virgin olive oil for flavor and texture.

7. Ground Cumin: 1/2 teaspoon of ground cumin adds a hint of warmth.

8. Paprika: 1/2 teaspoon of paprika for a smoky touch.

9. Salt and Pepper: Season the hummus with salt and freshly ground black pepper to taste.

For Garnish (Optional):

10. Fresh Parsley: Chopped fresh parsley or cilantro for garnish.

11. Olive Oil: Extra olive oil for drizzling on top.

Instructions:

1. Roast the Red Peppers:

Preheat your oven to 450°F (230°C). Place the whole red bell peppers on a baking sheet and roast them in the oven for about 20-25 minutes, turning occasionally, until the skins are charred and blistered. Remove them from the oven and let them cool.

2. Peel and Seed the Peppers:

Once the roasted red peppers have cooled enough to handle, peel off the charred skin and remove the seeds and stems. Cut the peppers into smaller pieces.

3. Prepare the Hummus:

In a food processor, combine the drained chickpeas, tahini, lemon juice, minced garlic, olive oil, ground cumin, paprika, salt, and black pepper.

4. Add Roasted Red Peppers:

Add the roasted red pepper pieces to the food processor.

5. Blend until Smooth:

Process the ingredients until the mixture becomes smooth and creamy. You may need to scrape down the sides of the food processor bowl and blend again for an even consistency.

6. Adjust Seasoning:

Taste the hummus and adjust the seasoning as needed. You can add more lemon juice, salt, or spices to suit your taste.

7. Garnish and Serve:

Transfer the roasted red pepper hummus to a serving bowl. If desired, drizzle with extra olive oil and garnish with chopped fresh parsley or cilantro.

8. Serve and Enjoy:

Your roasted red pepper hummus is ready to be enjoyed. Serve it as a dip with pita bread, carrot sticks, cucumber slices, or use it as a spread on sandwiches or wraps.

Tips:

If you're using jarred roasted red peppers, use about 1 cup of drained and chopped peppers.

For an extra-smooth hummus, you can peel the chickpeas by gently pinching them between your fingers to remove the skins before blending.

To control the thickness of the hummus, you can adjust the amount of olive oil and lemon juice. Add more for a smoother and thinner consistency, or reduce for a thicker dip.

Customize your roasted red pepper hummus by adding a pinch of red pepper flakes for some heat or a drizzle of balsamic vinegar for extra flavor.

Store leftover hummus in an airtight container in the refrigerator for up to a week. Drizzle a thin layer of olive oil on top to keep it fresh.

# Guacamole and Veggie Sticks

Guacamole and veggie sticks make for a delicious and healthy snack or appetizer. Guacamole is a creamy avocado-based dip that pairs perfectly with crunchy and fresh vegetable sticks. Here's a detailed guide on how to prepare guacamole and serve it with veggie sticks:

Ingredients:

For the Guacamole:

1. Avocados: You'll need 3 ripe avocados, peeled and pitted.

2. Lime Juice: Juice from 2 limes (about 2-3 tablespoons) for acidity and freshness.

3. Red Onion: 1/4 cup finely chopped red onion adds a mild oniony flavor.

4. Tomatoes: 2 Roma tomatoes, diced, for a juicy and slightly sweet element.

5. Jalapeño Pepper (Optional): Remove the seeds and finely chop a small jalapeño pepper for a hint of heat. Adjust the amount to your spice preference.

6. Fresh Cilantro: 1/4 cup chopped fresh cilantro adds a fresh and herbal note.

7. Garlic: One clove of garlic, minced, for savory depth.

8. Salt: About 1 teaspoon of salt, or to taste.

For the Veggie Sticks:

9. Vegetables: Choose a variety of fresh vegetables for dipping. Common choices include carrot sticks, cucumber slices, bell pepper strips (red, yellow, and green), celery sticks, and cherry tomatoes.

Instructions:

1. Prepare the Guacamole:

In a mixing bowl, mash the ripe avocados with a fork until they reach your desired level of creaminess. Some people prefer it slightly chunky, while others like it smoother.

2. Add Lime Juice:

Squeeze the juice from the limes into the mashed avocados. The acidity of the lime juice not only adds flavor but also prevents the avocados from browning.

3. Add Chopped Vegetables:

Add the finely chopped red onion, diced tomatoes, minced jalapeño pepper (if using), chopped cilantro, and minced garlic to the bowl with the mashed avocados.

4. Season with Salt:

Sprinkle about 1 teaspoon of salt over the guacamole mixture. You can adjust the salt to your taste.

5. Mix Well:

Gently fold all the ingredients together until well combined. Be careful not to overmix, as you want to maintain some texture in the guacamole.

6. Taste and Adjust:

Taste the guacamole and adjust the seasoning if needed. You can add more lime juice, salt, or even some additional chopped cilantro or jalapeño for extra flavor.

7. Prepare Veggie Sticks:

While making the guacamole, wash and prepare the vegetable sticks for dipping. Cut the vegetables into strips, slices, or sticks, depending on your preference.

8. Serve:

Transfer the guacamole to a serving bowl. Arrange the freshly cut veggie sticks on a platter or around the guacamole bowl.

9. Enjoy:

Your guacamole and veggie sticks are ready to be enjoyed. Dip the veggie sticks into the creamy guacamole for a satisfying and healthy snack.

Tips:

To prevent the guacamole from turning brown, place a piece of plastic wrap directly on the surface of the guacamole to minimize air exposure. Alternatively, squeeze extra lime juice on top and seal it with an airtight lid.

Customize your guacamole by adding ingredients like diced red or yellow bell peppers, diced red radishes, or even a touch of hot sauce for extra flavor.

If you like it spicier, leave some of the jalapeño seeds in or use a hotter pepper like serrano.

Serve the guacamole and veggie sticks immediately for the freshest experience, as avocados can brown over time.

You can also serve guacamole with tortilla chips for a different twist on this classic dip.

# Almond-Crusted Baked Chicken Tenders

Almond-crusted baked chicken tenders are a healthier alternative to traditional fried chicken tenders. They are crispy on the outside and tender on the inside, thanks to the nutty crunch of almond coating. Here's a detailed guide on how to make almond-crusted baked chicken tenders:

Ingredients:

For the Chicken Tenders:

1. Chicken Tenders: You'll need about 1.5 pounds (680 grams) of chicken tenders, which are boneless and skinless.

2. Almonds: 1 cup of whole almonds, unsalted and preferably raw.

3. Flour: 1/2 cup of all-purpose flour for dredging the chicken.

4. Eggs: 2 large eggs, beaten.

5. Olive Oil: 2 tablespoons of extra-virgin olive oil for coating the chicken.

6. Salt and Pepper: To season the chicken and the coating.

For the Coating:

7. Paprika: 1 teaspoon of paprika adds a smoky and slightly spicy flavor.

8. Garlic Powder: 1/2 teaspoon of garlic powder enhances the overall savory taste.

9. Onion Powder: 1/2 teaspoon of onion powder complements the other seasonings.

10. Dried Oregano (Optional): A pinch of dried oregano for extra flavor.

11. Parmesan Cheese (Optional): 1/4 cup of grated Parmesan cheese adds richness.

Instructions:

1. Preheat the Oven:

Preheat your oven to 425°F (220°C). Place a wire rack on a baking sheet and lightly grease it with cooking spray or olive oil.

2. Prepare the Almonds:

In a food processor, pulse the whole almonds until they are finely ground, resembling breadcrumbs. Be careful not to over-process, or they may turn into almond butter. Transfer the ground almonds to a shallow dish.

3. Prepare the Coating Mixture:

In another shallow dish, combine the flour, paprika, garlic powder, onion powder, dried oregano (if using), grated

Parmesan cheese (if using), salt, and pepper. Mix well to evenly distribute the seasonings.

4. Coat the Chicken:

Season the chicken tenders with salt and pepper. Dip each chicken tender into the flour mixture, ensuring it's evenly coated.

5. Dip in Eggs:

Next, dip the floured chicken tender into the beaten eggs, allowing any excess to drip off.

6. Coat with Almonds:

Roll the chicken tender in the ground almonds, pressing the almonds onto the chicken to create a coating. Place the coated chicken tender on the prepared wire rack on the baking sheet.

7. Repeat:

Repeat the process for all the chicken tenders, arranging them in a single layer on the wire rack.

8. Drizzle with Olive Oil:

Drizzle the tops of the almond-crusted chicken tenders with olive oil. This helps them become crispy during baking.

9. Bake:

Bake in the preheated oven for about 20-25 minutes or until the chicken is cooked through, and the almond coating is golden brown and crispy. The internal temperature of the chicken should reach 165°F (74°C).

10. Serve:

Once baked, remove the almond-crusted chicken tenders from the oven and let them cool for a minute or two. Serve them hot as an appetizer, main dish, or snack.

Tips:

Feel free to adjust the seasonings to your taste. You can add more or less paprika, garlic powder, or other seasonings to suit your preferences.

For extra flavor, you can add a pinch of cayenne pepper or smoked paprika to the coating mixture for a hint of heat and smokiness.

Serve the almond-crusted chicken tenders with your favorite dipping sauces, such as honey mustard, ranch, or barbecue sauce.

To make them gluten-free, you can use almond flour or gluten-free flour instead of all-purpose flour.

Store any leftovers in an airtight container in the refrigerator for up to 2-3 days and reheat them in the oven to maintain their crispiness.

# Chapter 6: Comforting Main Dishes

# Baked Salmon with Lemon-Dill Sauce

Baked salmon with lemon-dill sauce is a delightful and healthy dish that combines the rich, flaky texture of salmon with the fresh and zesty flavors of lemon and dill. This recipe is easy to prepare and perfect for a special dinner or a weeknight meal. Here's a detailed guide on how to make baked salmon with lemon-dill sauce:

Ingredients:

For the Baked Salmon:

1. Salmon Fillets: You'll need 4 salmon fillets, preferably skin-on, each about 6-8 ounces.

2. Olive Oil: 2 tablespoons of extra-virgin olive oil for brushing the salmon.

3. Salt and Pepper: To season the salmon fillets.

For the Lemon-Dill Sauce:

4. Fresh Lemon Juice: Juice from 2 lemons (about 1/4 cup) for a zesty kick.

5. Fresh Dill: 2-3 tablespoons of chopped fresh dill for a refreshing herbal flavor.

6. Garlic: Two cloves of garlic, minced, for savory depth.

7. Dijon Mustard: 1 teaspoon of Dijon mustard for a hint of tanginess.

8. Honey: 1 teaspoon of honey for sweetness (adjust to taste).

9. Salt and Pepper: To season the sauce.

Instructions:

1. Preheat the Oven:

Preheat your oven to 375°F (190°C). Line a baking sheet with parchment paper or lightly grease it.

2. Season the Salmon:

Place the salmon fillets on the prepared baking sheet, skin-side down. Brush the tops of the fillets with olive oil and season them generously with salt and pepper.

3. Bake the Salmon:

Bake the salmon in the preheated oven for about 12-15 minutes, or until the salmon flakes easily with a fork. The exact cooking time may vary depending on the thickness of the fillets. As a general rule, salmon should be cooked until it reaches an internal temperature of 145°F (63°C).

4. Prepare the Lemon-Dill Sauce:

While the salmon is baking, prepare the lemon-dill sauce. In a small bowl, whisk together the fresh lemon juice, chopped fresh dill, minced garlic, Dijon mustard, honey, salt, and pepper. Adjust the seasoning to taste.

5. Serve:

Once the salmon is done baking, remove it from the oven and let it rest for a few minutes. Carefully lift the salmon fillets off the skin if necessary.

6. Drizzle with Sauce:

Drizzle the lemon-dill sauce over the baked salmon fillets. You can also reserve some sauce to serve on the side.

7. Garnish:

Garnish the salmon with additional fresh dill and lemon slices if desired.

8. Serve and Enjoy:

Your baked salmon with lemon-dill sauce is ready to be served. It pairs well with a variety of side dishes, such as steamed vegetables, rice, or a fresh salad.

Tips:

To add an extra layer of flavor, you can marinate the salmon in the lemon-dill sauce for 15-30 minutes before baking. This will infuse the salmon with more flavor.

Ensure your salmon fillets are evenly sized to ensure even cooking. If some pieces are thicker than others, they may need a few extra minutes in the oven.

If you prefer your salmon skin crispy, you can broil the salmon for a minute or two after baking to crisp up the skin. Watch it carefully to avoid burning.

Feel free to customize the lemon-dill sauce by adding a pinch of red pepper flakes for a subtle heat or a touch of grated lemon zest for extra lemony flavor.

Store any leftover lemon-dill sauce in the refrigerator for up to a week and use it as a dressing for salads or as a sauce for other dishes.

# Grilled Vegetable and Quinoa Bowl

A grilled vegetable and quinoa bowl is a healthy and satisfying meal that's packed with flavors, nutrients, and textures. This dish combines the smokiness of grilled vegetables with the nutty goodness of quinoa, creating a balanced and hearty bowl. Here's a detailed guide on how to make a grilled vegetable and quinoa bowl:

Ingredients:

For the Grilled Vegetables:

1. Bell Peppers: Use a variety of bell peppers (red, yellow, and green), sliced into strips.

2. Zucchini: 2 medium-sized zucchinis, sliced into rounds.

3. Eggplant: 1 medium eggplant, sliced into rounds or strips.

4. Red Onion: 1 large red onion, sliced into rings.

5. Cherry Tomatoes: 1 cup of cherry tomatoes.

6. Olive Oil: 3-4 tablespoons of extra-virgin olive oil.

7. Balsamic Vinegar: 2 tablespoons of balsamic vinegar for added flavor.

8. Garlic: 2-3 cloves of garlic, minced.

9. Fresh Herbs: A handful of fresh herbs like basil, thyme, or rosemary, chopped.

10. Salt and Pepper: To season the vegetables.

For the Quinoa:

11. Quinoa: 1 cup of quinoa, rinsed.

12. Vegetable Broth or Water: 2 cups of vegetable broth or water for cooking the quinoa.

For the Lemon-Tahini Dressing:

13. Tahini: 1/4 cup of tahini paste.

14. Lemon Juice: Juice from 1 lemon (about 2-3 tablespoons).

15. Water: 2-4 tablespoons of water for thinning the dressing.

16. Garlic: 1 clove of garlic, minced.

17. Salt and Pepper: To season the dressing.

Instructions:

1. Prepare the Grilled Vegetables:

In a large bowl, combine the sliced bell peppers, zucchini, eggplant, red onion rings, and cherry tomatoes.

2. Prepare the Marinade:

In a separate bowl, whisk together the olive oil, balsamic vinegar, minced garlic, chopped fresh herbs, salt, and pepper.

3. Marinate the Vegetables:

Pour the marinade over the vegetables and toss to coat them evenly. Allow them to marinate for at least 15-30 minutes, allowing the flavors to meld.

4. Preheat the Grill:

Preheat your grill to medium-high heat. Make sure the grates are clean and lightly oiled to prevent sticking.

5. Grill the Vegetables:

Place the marinated vegetables on the grill and cook for about 3-5 minutes per side or until they have grill marks and are tender. Remove them from the grill and set aside.

6. Prepare the Quinoa:

In a medium saucepan, combine the rinsed quinoa and vegetable broth or water. Bring it to a boil, then reduce the heat to low, cover, and simmer for 15-20 minutes, or until the quinoa is cooked and the liquid is absorbed. Fluff the quinoa with a fork and set it aside.

7. Prepare the Lemon-Tahini Dressing:

In a small bowl, whisk together the tahini paste, lemon juice, minced garlic, and a pinch of salt and pepper. Add water, one tablespoon at a time, to achieve your desired dressing consistency. Taste and adjust the seasoning as needed.

8. Assemble the Bowl:

To assemble the grilled vegetable and quinoa bowl, start with a bed of cooked quinoa in each bowl. Top it with the grilled vegetables and cherry tomatoes.

9. Drizzle with Dressing:

Drizzle the lemon-tahini dressing generously over the vegetables and quinoa.

10. Garnish:

Garnish the bowls with additional fresh herbs, such as basil or thyme, and a sprinkle of salt and pepper if desired.

11. Serve and Enjoy:

Your grilled vegetable and quinoa bowl is ready to be served. Enjoy it as a wholesome and flavorful meal.

Tips:

Feel free to customize your grilled vegetable selection. You can add mushrooms, asparagus, or any of your favorite vegetables.

To save time, you can prepare the quinoa and lemon-tahini dressing while the vegetables are marinating or grilling.

If you don't have access to a grill, you can roast the marinated vegetables in the oven at 400°F (200°C) until they are tender and slightly caramelized.

Add some protein to your bowl by topping it with grilled chicken, tofu, chickpeas, or your preferred protein source.

Leftover grilled vegetables can be stored in the refrigerator and used in salads, sandwiches, or wraps. The lemon-tahini dressing also makes a great dip for raw veggies or a dressing for salads.

# Turmeric Chicken Curry

Turmeric chicken curry is a flavorful and aromatic dish that features tender chicken cooked in a rich and creamy sauce infused with the warm and earthy flavors of turmeric and other spices. Here's a detailed guide on how to make turmeric chicken curry:

Ingredients:

For the Curry:

1. Chicken: You'll need about 1.5 pounds (680 grams) of boneless, skinless chicken thighs or breasts, cut into bite-sized pieces.

2. Onion: 1 large onion, finely chopped.

3. Garlic: 4-5 cloves of garlic, minced.

4. Ginger: 1-inch piece of fresh ginger, grated or minced.

5. Tomatoes: 2 ripe tomatoes, finely chopped, or 1 can (14 ounces) of diced tomatoes.

6. Coconut Milk: 1 can (13.5 ounces) of full-fat coconut milk for creaminess.

7. Turmeric: 1 tablespoon of ground turmeric for the signature flavor and color.

8. Coriander Powder: 1 tablespoon of ground coriander.

9. Cumin Powder: 1 tablespoon of ground cumin.

10. Garam Masala: 1 teaspoon of garam masala for complexity and warmth.

11. Cayenne Pepper (Optional): A pinch of cayenne pepper for heat (adjust to your spice preference).

12. Salt and Pepper: To season the curry.

13. Cooking Oil: 2-3 tablespoons of cooking oil, such as vegetable oil or ghee.

For Garnish:

14. Fresh Cilantro: Chopped fresh cilantro leaves for garnish.

Instructions:

1. Prepare the Chicken:

Cut the chicken into bite-sized pieces and season them with salt and pepper. Set aside.

2. Sauté the Aromatics:

In a large skillet or saucepan, heat the cooking oil over medium heat. Add the chopped onion and sauté until it becomes translucent, about 5-7 minutes.

3. Add Garlic and Ginger:

Add the minced garlic and grated ginger to the sautéed onion. Cook for another 1-2 minutes until fragrant.

4. Spice it Up:

Stir in the ground turmeric, ground coriander, ground cumin, and a pinch of cayenne pepper (if using). Cook the spices with the aromatics for about a minute to release their flavors and aromas.

5. Add Tomatoes:

Add the finely chopped tomatoes (or canned diced tomatoes) to the pan. Cook for 5-7 minutes, or until the tomatoes break down and the mixture becomes somewhat thick.

6. Add Chicken:

Add the seasoned chicken pieces to the pan and stir to coat them with the tomato and spice mixture. Cook for about 5-7 minutes until the chicken starts to brown.

7. Coconut Milk:

Pour in the can of coconut milk, stirring to combine. Reduce the heat to low and simmer for about 15-20 minutes, or until the chicken is cooked through and the sauce thickens.

8. Season and Finish:

Season the curry with salt and pepper to taste. Add the
garam masala and stir it into the curry.

9. Garnish and Serve:

Once the chicken is fully cooked and the flavors have melded
together, remove the pan from heat. Garnish the turmeric
chicken curry with freshly chopped cilantro.

10. Serve and Enjoy:

Serve the turmeric chicken curry hot over steamed rice,
quinoa, or with naan bread for a complete and satisfying
meal.

Tips:

Customize the level of spiciness by adjusting the amount of
cayenne pepper or using fresh green chilies.

If you prefer a smoother sauce, you can blend the onion,
garlic, ginger, and tomato mixture before adding the chicken.

For extra creaminess, you can use a can of coconut cream
instead of coconut milk.

To add more vegetables to the curry, consider adding bell peppers, peas, or spinach during the last few minutes of cooking.

Leftover turmeric chicken curry can be refrigerated and reheated for another delicious meal the next day.

# Chapter 7: Sides and Accompaniments

## Garlic Mashed Cauliflower

Garlic mashed cauliflower is a low-carb and healthier alternative to traditional mashed potatoes. It's a creamy and flavorful side dish that's perfect for those looking to reduce their carb intake. Here's a detailed guide on how to make garlic mashed cauliflower:

Ingredients:

1. Cauliflower: You'll need one large head of cauliflower, trimmed and cut into florets.

2. Garlic: 3-4 cloves of garlic, minced.

3. Butter: 2-3 tablespoons of unsalted butter or olive oil for added richness.

4. Heavy Cream (Optional): 1/4 cup of heavy cream for extra creaminess (you can omit this for a lighter version).

5. Salt and Pepper: To season the mashed cauliflower.

6. Fresh Parsley (Optional): Chopped fresh parsley for garnish.

Instructions:

1. Prepare the Cauliflower:

Trim the cauliflower head and cut it into evenly sized florets. Discard the tough stem and leaves.

2. Steam the Cauliflower:

Place the cauliflower florets in a large steaming basket or a microwave-safe bowl. Steam the cauliflower until it is very tender, about 10-15 minutes. You can steam it on the stovetop or use a microwave.

3. Drain and Dry:

If there's any excess moisture after steaming, drain the cauliflower well. You want it to be as dry as possible to prevent a watery mashed consistency.

4. Mash the Cauliflower:

Transfer the steamed and drained cauliflower to a food processor or a large mixing bowl. Use a potato masher, hand blender, or a food processor to mash the cauliflower until it reaches your desired consistency. Some people prefer it slightly chunky, while others like it smoother.

5. Add Garlic:

While mashing the cauliflower, add the minced garlic. Continue to mash and mix until the garlic is evenly distributed.

6. Add Butter and Cream:

If you're using butter and heavy cream, add them to the mashed cauliflower. These ingredients add richness and creaminess to the dish. If you want a lighter version, you can omit the heavy cream and use olive oil instead of butter.

7. Season:

Season the garlic mashed cauliflower with salt and pepper to taste. Adjust the seasoning to your preference.

8. Taste and Adjust:

Taste the mashed cauliflower and adjust the seasoning if needed. You can add more minced garlic for a stronger garlic flavor or more butter and cream for richness.

9. Garnish:

If desired, garnish the garlic mashed cauliflower with chopped fresh parsley for a pop of color and freshness.

10. Serve and Enjoy:

Serve the garlic mashed cauliflower hot as a side dish. It pairs well with roasted meats, grilled chicken, or as a low-carb alternative to traditional mashed potatoes.

Tips:

For an even smoother consistency, you can use a hand blender or food processor to puree the mashed cauliflower.

To make it even more flavorful, you can add grated Parmesan cheese or a sprinkle of grated nutmeg.

If you prefer roasted garlic flavor, roast the garlic cloves in the oven with a little olive oil until they are soft and fragrant, then mash and add them to the cauliflower.

Store any leftovers in an airtight container in the refrigerator for up to 2-3 days. Reheat in the microwave or on the stovetop.

# Roasted Brussels Sprouts with Pecans

Roasted Brussels sprouts with pecans is a delightful side dish that combines the earthy flavors of Brussels sprouts with the nutty crunch of pecans. The roasting process enhances the natural sweetness of the sprouts while adding a crispy texture. Here's a detailed guide on how to make roasted Brussels sprouts with pecans:

Ingredients:

1. Brussels Sprouts: You'll need about 1.5 pounds (680 grams) of fresh Brussels sprouts, trimmed and halved.

2. Pecans: 1/2 cup of pecan halves or pieces.

3. Olive Oil: 2-3 tablespoons of extra-virgin olive oil for roasting.

4. Balsamic Vinegar (Optional): 2 tablespoons of balsamic vinegar for added flavor.

5. Garlic: 2-3 cloves of garlic, minced.

6. Honey (Optional): 1-2 tablespoons of honey for a touch of sweetness (adjust to taste).

7. Salt and Pepper: To season the Brussels sprouts.

Instructions:

1. Prepare the Brussels Sprouts:

Start by trimming the ends of the Brussels sprouts and removing any yellow or wilted outer leaves. Cut them in half lengthwise for even cooking.

2. Preheat the Oven:

Preheat your oven to 400°F (200°C). Place a rimmed baking sheet in the oven while it preheats.

3. Toss with Olive Oil:

In a large mixing bowl, toss the halved Brussels sprouts with the olive oil until they are evenly coated. Season with salt and pepper to taste.

4. Roast the Brussels Sprouts:

Carefully remove the hot baking sheet from the oven and spread the seasoned Brussels sprouts in a single layer. Roast in the preheated oven for about 20-25 minutes or until the sprouts are tender and golden brown, turning them halfway through for even cooking.

5. Add Pecans:

About halfway through the roasting time, add the pecan halves or pieces to the baking sheet with the partially roasted Brussels sprouts. This allows the pecans to become toasted and fragrant.

6. Prepare the Glaze (Optional):

While the Brussels sprouts are roasting, you can prepare a glaze if desired. In a small saucepan, combine the balsamic vinegar, minced garlic, and honey (if using). Heat the mixture over low heat, stirring until it thickens slightly. Remove it from heat.

7. Glaze and Serve:

Once the Brussels sprouts and pecans are done roasting, remove them from the oven. If you made the glaze, drizzle it over the roasted Brussels sprouts and pecans, tossing gently to coat.

8. Serve and Enjoy:

Transfer the roasted Brussels sprouts with pecans to a serving platter and serve hot. They make a wonderful side dish for various main courses, such as roasted chicken, grilled steak, or as a vegetarian option.

Tips:

Feel free to customize the seasoning by adding other herbs and spices like thyme, rosemary, or red pepper flakes for a kick of heat.

You can also experiment with different nuts like walnuts or almonds for a unique flavor and texture.

To make this dish vegan, omit the honey from the glaze or replace it with a vegan sweetener like maple syrup or agave nectar.

For a bit of tanginess, you can sprinkle freshly grated Parmesan cheese over the roasted Brussels sprouts just before serving.

Leftover roasted Brussels sprouts with pecans can be stored in an airtight container in the refrigerator for up to 3-4 days and reheated in the oven or microwave.

# Cucumber and Mint Yogurt Sauce

Cucumber and mint yogurt sauce, also known as tzatziki, is a refreshing and creamy condiment that pairs well with a variety of dishes. It's commonly used in Mediterranean and Middle Eastern cuisine to complement grilled meats, kebabs, falafel, or as a dip for pita bread and vegetables. Here's a detailed guide on how to make cucumber and mint yogurt sauce:

Ingredients:

1. Greek Yogurt: You'll need 1.5 cups (360 grams) of Greek yogurt, which is thicker and creamier than regular yogurt.

2. Cucumber: 1 medium cucumber, peeled, seeded, and finely grated.

3. Fresh Mint: 2-3 tablespoons of fresh mint leaves, finely chopped.

4. Garlic: 2-3 cloves of garlic, minced or finely grated.

5. Lemon Juice: Juice from 1 lemon (about 2-3 tablespoons).

6. Olive Oil: 1-2 tablespoons of extra-virgin olive oil.

7. Salt and Pepper: To season the sauce.

Instructions:

1. Prepare the Cucumber:

Start by peeling the cucumber, as the skin can be bitter. Cut the cucumber in half lengthwise and use a spoon to scoop out the seeds. Grate the cucumber using the fine side of a grater.

2. Drain the Cucumber:

Place the grated cucumber in a fine-mesh sieve or a clean kitchen towel. Squeeze out any excess moisture from the cucumber. This step is crucial to prevent the sauce from becoming too watery.

3. Mix Yogurt and Lemon Juice:

In a mixing bowl, combine the Greek yogurt and lemon juice. Stir well to incorporate the lemon juice into the yogurt.

4. Add Garlic:

Add the minced or grated garlic to the yogurt mixture. Garlic adds a robust flavor to the sauce, so you can adjust the amount to your preference.

5. Incorporate Grated Cucumber:

Gently fold the drained, grated cucumber into the yogurt mixture. This adds a refreshing crunch to the sauce.

6. Add Fresh Mint:

Chop the fresh mint leaves finely and add them to the sauce. Mint provides a pleasant herbal aroma and a burst of freshness.

7. Season with Olive Oil and Seasonings:

Drizzle the extra-virgin olive oil over the sauce and season with salt and pepper to taste. Mix everything together until well combined.

8. Refrigerate:

Cover the cucumber and mint yogurt sauce and refrigerate it for at least 30 minutes before serving. This allows the flavors to meld together and enhances the taste.

9. Serve and Enjoy:

Serve the cucumber and mint yogurt sauce chilled. It's a versatile condiment that pairs wonderfully with grilled meats, vegetables, pita bread, falafel, gyros, or as a dip for fresh vegetables.

Tips:

If you prefer a smoother sauce, you can blend the cucumber and mint yogurt sauce in a food processor or blender until you achieve your desired consistency.

Adjust the amount of garlic and mint based on your taste preferences. You can also experiment with other herbs like dill or parsley.

To make the sauce even creamier, you can use full-fat Greek yogurt.

If you want a dairy-free version, you can substitute the Greek yogurt with dairy-free yogurt alternatives like coconut yogurt or almond yogurt.

Leftover cucumber and mint yogurt sauce can be stored in an airtight container in the refrigerator for up to 2-3 days. Stir it well before serving any leftovers.

# Chapter 8: Desserts for Treat Days

## Blueberry Chia Seed Pudding

Blueberry chia seed pudding is a nutritious and delicious breakfast or snack option. It combines the goodness of chia seeds with the sweet and tangy flavor of blueberries, creating a creamy and satisfying pudding. Here's a detailed guide on how to make blueberry chia seed pudding:

Ingredients:

For the Blueberry Compote:

1. Blueberries: 1 cup of fresh or frozen blueberries.

2. Maple Syrup (or Honey): 2-3 tablespoons of maple syrup (adjust to taste) or honey.

3. Lemon Juice: Juice from half a lemon for a hint of tartness (optional).

For the Chia Seed Pudding:

4. Chia Seeds: 1/3 cup of chia seeds.

5. Greek Yogurt: 1 cup of Greek yogurt for creaminess.

6. Milk: 1.5 cups of milk (dairy or non-dairy, like almond or coconut milk).

7. Vanilla Extract: 1 teaspoon of vanilla extract for flavor.

8. Maple Syrup (or Honey): 2-3 tablespoons of maple syrup or honey (adjust to taste).

Instructions:

1. Prepare the Blueberry Compote:

In a saucepan, combine the blueberries and maple syrup (or honey). You can also add a splash of lemon juice for a hint of tartness. Cook the mixture over medium heat, stirring occasionally, until the blueberries break down and the sauce thickens, which takes about 10-15 minutes. Once done, remove it from heat and let it cool.

2. Make the Chia Seed Pudding Base:

In a mixing bowl, combine the chia seeds, Greek yogurt, milk, vanilla extract, and maple syrup (or honey). Stir everything together until well combined. Make sure the chia seeds are evenly distributed.

3. Let it Sit:

Cover the chia seed pudding mixture and refrigerate it for at least 30 minutes. This allows the chia seeds to absorb the liquid and create a pudding-like consistency. You can also refrigerate it overnight for a thicker texture.

4. Layer the Pudding:

Once the chia seed pudding has set, you can start layering it with the blueberry compote. You can use jars, glasses, or bowls for serving.

5. Layering:

Begin by spooning a layer of the chia seed pudding into each serving container. Next, add a layer of the blueberry compote on top of the pudding.

6. Repeat:

Continue to alternate layers of chia seed pudding and blueberry compote until you reach the desired number of layers. Finish with a spoonful of blueberry compote on top.

7. Garnish (Optional):

If desired, you can garnish the blueberry chia seed pudding with a few fresh blueberries, a drizzle of maple syrup, or a sprinkle of chopped nuts.

8. Serve and Enjoy:

Serve the blueberry chia seed pudding immediately or refrigerate it until you're ready to enjoy. It's a nutritious and satisfying breakfast, snack, or dessert option.

Tips:

Adjust the sweetness to your preference by adding more or less maple syrup or honey to both the blueberry compote and the chia seed pudding base.

Feel free to customize the layers by adding other fruits like strawberries, raspberries, or sliced bananas.

Chia seed pudding can be made ahead of time and stored in the refrigerator for up to 3-4 days. Keep it covered to maintain freshness.

Experiment with different flavors by adding spices like cinnamon or nutmeg to the chia seed pudding base.

This recipe is highly versatile, and you can use other berries or fruit compotes of your choice to create various flavors of chia seed pudding.

# Chocolate Avocado Mousse

Chocolate avocado mousse is a rich and creamy dessert that combines the indulgence of chocolate with the healthy goodness of avocados. It's a great way to satisfy your sweet tooth while also enjoying the benefits of nutrient-dense avocados. Here's a detailed guide on how to make chocolate avocado mousse:

Ingredients:

1. Ripe Avocados: You'll need 2 ripe avocados, peeled and pitted.

2. Cocoa Powder: 1/2 cup of unsweetened cocoa powder.

3. Maple Syrup (or Honey): 1/4 cup of pure maple syrup or honey (adjust to taste).

4. Vanilla Extract: 1 teaspoon of pure vanilla extract.

5. Salt: A pinch of salt to enhance the chocolate flavor.

6. Milk: 1/4 cup of milk (dairy or non-dairy, like almond milk or coconut milk).

7. Dark Chocolate (Optional): 2 ounces of melted dark chocolate for extra richness (70% cocoa or higher).

8. Toppings (Optional): Fresh berries, whipped cream, chopped nuts, or grated chocolate for garnish.

Instructions:

1. Prepare the Avocados:

Cut the ripe avocados in half, remove the pits, and scoop the flesh into a blender or food processor. Make sure the avocados are ripe and creamy for the best texture.

2. Add Cocoa Powder:

Add the unsweetened cocoa powder to the blender or food processor with the avocado.

3. Sweeten the Mixture:

Pour in the maple syrup (or honey) for sweetness, along with the vanilla extract and a pinch of salt. Adjust the sweetness to your taste preferences.

4. Blend Until Smooth:

Blend or process the mixture until it becomes smooth and creamy. You may need to stop and scrape down the sides of the blender or food processor to ensure everything is well combined.

5. Add Milk:

With the blender or food processor running, gradually add the milk (dairy or non-dairy) to achieve your desired mousse consistency. You can adjust the amount of milk based on how thick or creamy you want it.

6. Incorporate Melted Chocolate (Optional):

If you want an even richer chocolate flavor, you can add melted dark chocolate to the mixture. Simply melt the dark chocolate in the microwave or using a double boiler and pour it into the blender or food processor while it's running. Blend until well combined.

7. Taste and Adjust:

Taste the chocolate avocado mousse and adjust the sweetness or chocolate flavor as needed. You can add more maple syrup, cocoa powder, or melted chocolate if desired.

8. Chill:

Transfer the chocolate avocado mousse to serving dishes or glasses and refrigerate for at least 30 minutes to chill and set.

9. Serve and Garnish:

Serve the chilled chocolate avocado mousse with your choice of toppings, such as fresh berries, a dollop of whipped cream, chopped nuts, or grated chocolate.

10. Enjoy:

Enjoy your homemade chocolate avocado mousse as a decadent and healthier dessert option.

Tips:

Make sure the avocados are ripe but not overripe; they should be creamy and free of brown spots for the best texture and flavor.

For a smoother consistency, you can pass the mousse through a fine-mesh sieve to remove any remaining avocado fibers.

Feel free to customize the sweetness level to suit your taste. You can use more or less maple syrup or honey.

If you prefer a dairy-free version, use a non-dairy milk option and dairy-free dark chocolate.

Leftover chocolate avocado mousse can be stored in an airtight container in the refrigerator

# Mixed Berry Sorbet

Mixed berry sorbet is a delightful and refreshing frozen dessert made from a blend of various berries. It's a perfect way to enjoy the natural sweetness and vibrant flavors of fresh or frozen berries. Here's a detailed guide on how to make mixed berry sorbet:

Ingredients:

1. Mixed Berries: You'll need a total of 4 cups of mixed berries. You can use a combination of strawberries, blueberries, raspberries, and blackberries. Fresh or frozen berries work well.

2. Sugar: 1/2 to 3/4 cup of granulated sugar, depending on the sweetness of your berries and your taste preference.

3. Lemon Juice: Juice from 1 lemon (about 2-3 tablespoons).

4. Water: 1/4 cup of water.

Instructions:

1. Prepare the Berries:

If using fresh berries, wash them thoroughly and remove any stems or hulls. If using frozen berries, make sure they are properly thawed.

2. Blend the Berries:

Place the mixed berries in a blender or food processor. Add the lemon juice and blend until the berries are pureed and smooth.

3. Strain the Puree (Optional):

If you prefer a smoother sorbet without seeds, you can strain the berry puree through a fine-mesh sieve to remove any seeds. Use a spoon to press the puree through the sieve into a clean bowl.

4. Make the Simple Syrup:

In a small saucepan, combine the sugar and water. Heat over medium heat, stirring constantly, until the sugar completely dissolves. Remove from heat and let the simple syrup cool to room temperature.

5. Combine Syrup and Berry Puree:

Pour the cooled simple syrup into the berry puree and mix well to combine. Taste the mixture and adjust the sweetness by adding more sugar if needed.

6. Chill the Mixture:

Cover the berry mixture and refrigerate it for at least 2 hours or until it's thoroughly chilled. Chilling helps the sorbet freeze faster.

7. Freeze the Sorbet:

Pour the chilled berry mixture into an ice cream maker and churn according to the manufacturer's instructions. The sorbet will become thicker and freeze as it churns.

8. Transfer to a Container:

Once the sorbet reaches the desired consistency, transfer it to an airtight container.

9. Further Harden (Optional):

For a firmer sorbet, place the container in the freezer for an additional 2-3 hours or until the sorbet is solidified to your liking.

10. Serve and Enjoy:

Scoop the mixed berry sorbet into serving dishes or cones. Garnish with fresh berries or a mint sprig if desired. Enjoy the refreshing and fruity treat!

Tips:

You can customize the sweetness of the sorbet by adjusting the amount of sugar according to your taste.

If you don't have an ice cream maker, you can pour the mixture into a shallow, freezer-safe container, cover it, and freeze it. Every 30 minutes, stir the mixture with a fork to break up ice crystals until it reaches the desired consistency.

Feel free to experiment with other berry combinations or add a splash of liqueur like Chambord for an adult twist.

Leftover sorbet can be stored in an airtight container in the freezer for several weeks. Let it sit at room temperature for a few minutes to soften before scooping.

# Chapter 9: Beverages and Smoothies

# Ginger Turmeric Tea

Ginger turmeric tea is a warming and soothing beverage that combines the earthy spiciness of ginger with the anti-inflammatory properties of turmeric. It's not only delicious but also packed with health benefits. Here's a detailed guide on how to make ginger turmeric tea:

Ingredients:

1. Fresh Ginger: A 2-inch piece of fresh ginger root, peeled and thinly sliced, or 2 tablespoons of grated ginger.

2. Turmeric: 1 teaspoon of ground turmeric or a 1-inch piece of fresh turmeric root, thinly sliced.

3. Water: 4 cups of water.

4. Lemon (Optional): Slices or juice from 1 lemon.

5. Honey (Optional): 2-3 tablespoons of honey for sweetness (adjust to taste).

Instructions:

1. Prepare the Ginger and Turmeric:

If using fresh ginger and turmeric, peel and thinly slice them or grate them using a fine grater.

2. Boil the Water:

In a medium-sized saucepan, bring 4 cups of water to a boil.

3. Add Ginger and Turmeric:

Once the water is boiling, add the sliced or grated ginger and turmeric to the saucepan.

4. Simmer:

Reduce the heat to low, cover the saucepan, and let the mixture simmer for about 10-15 minutes. Simmering allows the ginger and turmeric to infuse the water with their flavors and beneficial compounds.

5. Strain:

After simmering, remove the saucepan from heat and strain the tea through a fine-mesh sieve or a tea strainer into a teapot or serving cups.

6. Add Lemon and Honey (Optional):

If desired, you can add slices of lemon or a squeeze of lemon juice for a hint of citrusy freshness. You can also sweeten the tea with honey if you prefer a sweeter taste.

7. Serve and Enjoy:

Serve the ginger turmeric tea hot and savor its soothing warmth and comforting flavor.

Tips:

Adjust the amount of ginger, turmeric, lemon, and honey to suit your taste preferences. Some people prefer a stronger ginger or turmeric flavor, while others like it milder.

You can use a tea infuser or a muslin bag to contain the ginger and turmeric during simmering, making it easier to strain later.

Fresh turmeric root is available in some grocery stores and can be used in place of ground turmeric for a more intense flavor and color.

This tea is known for its potential health benefits, including anti-inflammatory properties and digestive aid. However, it's always a good idea to consult with a healthcare professional if you have any specific health concerns or are taking medications.

You can enjoy ginger turmeric tea as is, or you can customize it by adding other spices like cinnamon or black pepper for extra flavor and health benefits.

Store any leftover tea in the refrigerator and reheat it as needed. It can be enjoyed both hot and cold.

# Pineapple and Spinach Smoothie

A pineapple and spinach smoothie is a vibrant and nutritious beverage that combines the tropical sweetness of pineapple with the health benefits of spinach. It's a great way to sneak in some leafy greens into your diet while enjoying a refreshing drink. Here's a detailed guide on how to make a pineapple and spinach smoothie:

Ingredients:

1. Pineapple: 1 cup of fresh pineapple chunks or 1/2 cup of canned pineapple chunks (packed in juice, not syrup).

2. Spinach: 2 cups of fresh spinach leaves, tightly packed.

3. Banana: 1 ripe banana, peeled and sliced.

4. Greek Yogurt: 1/2 cup of plain Greek yogurt for creaminess.

5. Orange Juice: 1/2 cup of fresh orange juice for a citrusy kick.

6. Water (Optional): 1/4 cup of water to adjust the consistency (add more if needed).

7. Honey or Maple Syrup (Optional): 1-2 tablespoons for added sweetness (adjust to taste).

Instructions:

1. Prepare the Ingredients:

Peel and slice the ripe banana. If you're using fresh pineapple, peel and cut it into chunks. Make sure to remove any tough core pieces.

2. Blend the Spinach:

Start by blending the spinach with the orange juice until it's well blended and you have a green liquid.

3. Add the Remaining Ingredients:

Add the pineapple chunks, sliced banana, Greek yogurt, and honey or maple syrup (if using) to the blender.

4. Blend Until Smooth:

Blend all the ingredients together until the mixture is smooth and creamy. If the smoothie is too thick, you can add a little water to reach your desired consistency.

5. Taste and Adjust:

Taste the smoothie and adjust the sweetness by adding more honey or maple syrup if needed.

6. Serve and Enjoy:

Pour the pineapple and spinach smoothie into a glass and enjoy it as a nutritious and refreshing snack or breakfast.

Tips:

Feel free to customize this smoothie by adding other ingredients like chia seeds, flaxseeds, or protein powder for an extra nutritional boost.

If you prefer a colder smoothie, you can add ice cubes to the blender while blending.

For a dairy-free version, you can use coconut yogurt or almond milk yogurt instead of Greek yogurt.

Experiment with the sweetness level by adjusting the amount of honey or maple syrup. You can also make it completely sugar-free if your fruits are sweet enough.

This smoothie can be a great way to introduce more greens into your diet, especially if you have picky eaters at home who might not enjoy eating spinach on its own.

Pineapple and spinach are both excellent sources of vitamins and antioxidants, making this smoothie a healthy choice.

# Anti-Inflammatory Golden Milk

Anti-inflammatory golden milk, also known as turmeric milk or "haldi doodh" in some cultures, is a warm and comforting beverage renowned for its potential health benefits. This soothing elixir combines the vibrant yellow spice turmeric with other ingredients like milk, spices, and sweeteners to create a delicious and wellness-boosting drink. Here's a detailed guide on how to make anti-inflammatory golden milk:

Ingredients:

1. Turmeric: 1 teaspoon of ground turmeric or a 1-inch piece of fresh turmeric root, thinly sliced.

2. Milk: 1 cup of your choice of milk (dairy or non-dairy, such as almond, coconut, or oat milk).

3. Sweetener: 1-2 tablespoons of honey, maple syrup, or a sweetener of your choice (adjust to taste).

4. Spices: A pinch of black pepper (enhances the absorption of curcumin, the active compound in turmeric), a pinch of ground cinnamon, a pinch of ground ginger (optional).

5. Fat (Optional): 1 teaspoon of coconut oil or ghee (clarified butter) to enhance the absorption of curcumin.

Instructions:

1. Prepare the Turmeric:

If using fresh turmeric root, peel and thinly slice it. If using ground turmeric, measure out 1 teaspoon.

2. Heat the Milk:

In a small saucepan, heat the milk over medium heat until it's steaming but not boiling. Stir occasionally to prevent sticking or scorching.

3. Add Turmeric and Spices:

Reduce the heat to low and add the ground turmeric (or fresh turmeric slices) and spices (black pepper, ground cinnamon, and ground ginger) to the milk. Stir well to combine.

4. Simmer:

Allow the mixture to simmer on low heat for about 5-10 minutes. This simmering infuses the milk with the flavors of the spices and turmeric.

5. Add Sweetener:

After simmering, remove the saucepan from heat and add your preferred sweetener (honey, maple syrup, etc.). Adjust the sweetness to your taste.

6. Include Fat (Optional):

If desired, stir in 1 teaspoon of coconut oil or ghee to enhance the absorption of curcumin. This step is optional but recommended for better absorption of turmeric's health benefits.

7. Strain and Serve:

If you used fresh turmeric slices, strain the golden milk through a fine-mesh sieve or tea strainer to remove the solids. Pour the strained golden milk into a cup or mug.

8. Enjoy Warm:

Sip your anti-inflammatory golden milk while it's still warm and comforting. Feel free to garnish with a sprinkle of ground cinnamon or a cinnamon stick for extra flavor and presentation.

Tips:

Adjust the amount of sweetener and spices to suit your taste preferences. Some people prefer a stronger ginger or cinnamon flavor, while others like it milder.

Fresh turmeric root can be found in some grocery stores or specialty markets. If using it, be cautious, as it can stain surfaces and clothing.

You can prepare a larger batch of golden milk and refrigerate it for later use. Reheat gently on the stove or in the microwave when ready to enjoy.

Turmeric is renowned for its potential anti-inflammatory and antioxidant properties. However, it's essential to consult with a healthcare professional before incorporating it into your diet, especially if you have any specific health concerns or are taking medications.

Golden milk is not only comforting but also a great way to incorporate the potential health benefits of turmeric into your daily routine. Enjoy it as a soothing bedtime drink or a warm pick-me-up during the day.

# Chapter 10: Meal Plans and Tips

## Weekly Meal Plans

Weekly meal planning is a systematic approach to organizing your meals and snacks for an entire week. This process helps you make informed dietary choices, save time and money, reduce food waste, and maintain a healthier lifestyle. Here's a detailed guide on creating weekly meal plans:

1. Set Clear Goals:

Begin by defining your meal planning goals. Are you aiming to eat healthier, save time on cooking, or reduce food expenses? Having clear objectives will guide your planning process.

2. Choose a Planning Tool:

Select a method for creating and recording your meal plan. Options include digital apps, meal planning templates, notebooks, or a whiteboard in your kitchen.

3. Inventory Your Kitchen:

Before planning, take stock of what you have in your pantry, fridge, and freezer. This prevents buying duplicates and helps you incorporate existing ingredients into your meals.

4. Consider Dietary Needs:

Factor in dietary restrictions or preferences, such as vegetarian, vegan, gluten-free, or any allergies or intolerances, when planning your meals.

5. Create a Weekly Calendar:

Set up a calendar for the week, including all meals (breakfast, lunch, dinner), snacks, and any special occasions or events that may affect your meal choices.

6. Plan for Balance:

Ensure each meal includes a balance of macronutrients (carbohydrates, proteins, and fats) and incorporates a variety of colorful fruits and vegetables. Include whole grains and lean proteins.

7. Rotate Proteins:

Avoid eating the same protein source every day. Rotate between poultry, fish, beans, lentils, tofu, and other protein-rich foods for variety.

8. Plan Leftovers:

Strategically plan for leftovers, especially for dinner, to reduce cooking time and food waste. Cook extra portions that can serve as the next day's lunch or dinner.

9. Incorporate Seasonal Produce:

Use seasonal fruits and vegetables in your meal plan. Not only are they fresher, but they are often more affordable and environmentally friendly.

10. Recipe Selection:

- Choose recipes based on your meal plan. Be sure to include dishes you enjoy, new recipes you want to try, and easy-to-prep meals for busy days.

11. Grocery List:

- As you plan your meals, create a corresponding grocery list. Organize it by categories (e.g., produce, dairy, pantry) to make shopping efficient.

12. Prep Ahead:

- Dedicate time for meal prep. Chop vegetables, marinate proteins, and prepare grains or sauces in advance to streamline cooking during the week.

13. Theme Nights:

- Assign theme nights to add variety and structure to your plan. For example, "Meatless Monday" or "Taco Tuesday" can make planning more fun.

14. Flexibility:

- Allow flexibility in your plan for unforeseen circumstances. Include "leftover nights" or simpler options for days when cooking isn't feasible.

15. Portion Control:

- Be mindful of portion sizes to prevent overeating. Use measuring cups and scales if necessary, especially when tracking calories or specific nutrients.

16. Review and Adjust:

- Periodically assess your meal plan's effectiveness. Adjust it based on your goals, dietary preferences, and feedback from family members.

17. Record and Reflect:

- Keep a journal or record of your meal plans, noting what worked well and what didn't. Use this information to refine future plans and improve your eating habits.

18. Shop Wisely:

- Stick to your grocery list, avoid impulse purchases, and consider buying in bulk for non-perishable items to save money.

19. Enjoy the Process:

- Embrace meal planning as a creative and enjoyable activity. Involve family members in the planning process to cater to their preferences.

20. Celebrate Successes:

- Acknowledge the benefits of meal planning, such as healthier eating habits, reduced food waste, and the convenience of having prepped meals. Celebrate your achievements.


Weekly meal planning is a valuable tool for achieving your dietary and lifestyle goals. It helps you take control of your nutrition, streamline your cooking routine, and enjoy balanced, satisfying meals throughout the week. Whether you're a busy professional, a parent, or simply looking to make better food choices, a well-structured meal plan can simplify your life and contribute to your overall well-being.

# Grocery Shopping Guide

Creating a grocery shopping guide is an excellent way to plan your meals, save money, and make healthier food choices. Here's a detailed guide on how to create an effective grocery shopping list:

1. Plan Your Meals:

Before you start making a shopping list, plan your meals for the week. Think about breakfast, lunch, dinner, and any snacks you'll need. Consider dietary restrictions and preferences.

2. Take Inventory:

Check your pantry, refrigerator, and freezer to see what ingredients you already have. This prevents buying duplicates and helps you use up items before they expire.

3. Categorize Your List:

Divide your shopping list into categories like produce, dairy, meat, pantry staples, and household items. This organization makes shopping more efficient.

4. Prioritize Nutrient-Rich Foods:

Focus on purchasing fresh fruits, vegetables, whole grains, lean proteins, and healthy fats. Minimize processed foods and sugary snacks.

5. Include Staples:

Ensure your pantry is stocked with essential staples like rice, pasta, canned tomatoes, beans, cooking oils, and spices.

6. Consider Batch Cooking:

Plan for batch cooking and meal prep. Buy ingredients in bulk if you intend to prepare meals in advance.

7. Check Sales and Discounts:

Look for sales, discounts, and coupons in your local grocery store's flyer or online. Take advantage of these deals when they align with your shopping list.

8. Stick to Your Budget:

Set a budget for your shopping trip and stick to it. Avoid impulse purchases that can add up quickly.

9. Buy Seasonal Produce:

Choose seasonal fruits and vegetables, as they are often fresher and more affordable. Plus, they add variety to your meals throughout the year.

10. Consider Frozen and Canned Options:

- Include frozen fruits and vegetables or canned goods like beans and tomatoes, which have a longer shelf life and can be used in a pinch.

11. Think About Beverages:

- Include drinks like water, milk, or herbal tea on your list. Minimize sugary drinks and excessive alcoholic beverages.

12. Don't Forget Snacks:

- If you enjoy snacks, include healthier options like nuts, yogurt, or cut-up vegetables. Limit the availability of less healthy snacks.

13. Include Household Items:

- If you need non-food items like cleaning supplies or toiletries, add them to your list so you can get everything in one trip.

## 14. Be Mindful of Expiry Dates:

- Check the expiry dates on perishable items, especially dairy, meat, and packaged goods. Buy quantities that you can consume before they expire.

## 15. Reusable Bags and List:

- Bring reusable shopping bags to reduce plastic waste and use a digital or paper list to stay organized.

## 16. Review Your List:

- Before heading to the store, review your list one more time to ensure you haven't missed anything important.

## 17. Stick to the List:

- While shopping, resist the urge to deviate from your list unless you come across a truly exceptional deal or a necessary substitution.

## 18. Check for Freshness:

- Inspect fresh produce, meat, and dairy items for freshness and quality. Choose items with the longest shelf life when possible.

19. Stay Organized in the Store:

- Navigate the store efficiently by following the categories on your list. This prevents backtracking and saves time.

20. Be Mindful of Portions:

- Avoid buying excessively large portions, especially for perishable items, unless you plan to freeze or use them promptly.

Creating a well-organized grocery shopping guide helps streamline your shopping trips, reduces food waste, and supports healthier eating habits. It also helps you maintain control over your food budget and make more informed food choices.

# Arthritis-Friendly Cooking Tips

Arthritis-friendly cooking tips can make meal preparation more manageable and enjoyable for individuals with arthritis, a condition that can cause joint pain, stiffness, and reduced mobility. These tips focus on creating a kitchen environment and cooking techniques that minimize stress on the joints and maximize ease and comfort. Here are detailed arthritis-friendly cooking tips:

1. Ergonomic Kitchen Tools:

Invest in ergonomic kitchen utensils and tools designed to reduce strain on the hands and joints. Look for utensils with padded handles, larger grips, and lightweight materials.

2. Electric Appliances:

Consider using electric appliances like an electric can opener, food processor, and electric kettle. These can make tasks like chopping, opening cans, and boiling water much easier.

3. Sharp Knives:

Keep your knives sharp. Dull knives require more force to cut, increasing the risk of strain. Use a knife sharpener or have your knives professionally sharpened.

4. Pre-Cut Ingredients:

Purchase pre-cut or pre-chopped vegetables and fruits when available. This saves time and minimizes the need for repetitive cutting and chopping.

5. Kitchen Organization:

Keep your kitchen organized. Store frequently used items within easy reach, eliminating the need to stretch or bend excessively. Consider pull-out shelves or lazy Susans in cabinets.

6. Anti-Fatigue Mats:

Use anti-fatigue mats in areas where you stand for extended periods, such as in front of the sink or stove. These mats provide cushioning and reduce joint stress.

7. Stovetop Control Knobs:

Replace traditional stove control knobs with larger, easier-to-grip knobs or consider getting a stove with front-mounted controls.

8. Use Utensils:

Use utensils like tongs or a Reacher/grabber to access items on high shelves or in deep cabinets. Avoid overstretching or climbing on stools.

9. Slow Cooking and Pressure Cooking:

Consider using slow cookers or pressure cookers for one-pot meals. These appliances require minimal stirring and reduce the need for constant attention.

10. Batch Cooking:

- Prepare larger batches of meals and freeze portions for later use. This reduces the frequency of cooking and allows you to have readily available, arthritis-friendly meals.

11. Assistive Devices:

- Explore assistive devices like jar openers, bottle openers, and easy-to-use can openers designed for individuals with limited hand strength.

12. Seating:

- If possible, use a chair or stool with back support while cooking. This allows you to sit when performing tasks that don't require standing.

13. Adaptive Techniques:

- Learn adaptive cooking techniques, such as using a two-handed rolling pin or adaptive cutting boards that hold food in place.

14. Avoid Excess Salt:

- Minimize the use of excess salt in your cooking, as excessive salt intake can exacerbate inflammation associated with arthritis.

15. Foods for Joint Health:

- Include foods rich in omega-3 fatty acids (like fatty fish), antioxidants (like berries and leafy greens), and anti-inflammatory spices (like turmeric and ginger) in your diet for joint health.

16. Stay Hydrated:

- Drink plenty of water throughout the day to keep your joints lubricated. Proper hydration is essential for overall joint health.

## 17. Moderate Portions:

- Practice portion control to maintain a healthy weight. Excess weight can put added stress on joints, especially those in the lower body.

## 18. Stay Active:

- Engage in gentle, low-impact exercises to maintain joint flexibility and muscle strength. Consult a physical therapist for tailored exercises.

## 19. Pace Yourself:

- Take breaks when needed and avoid overexertion. Listen to your body and rest when fatigue or discomfort sets in.

## 20. Consult a Dietitian:

- Consider consulting a dietitian or nutritionist specializing in arthritis or inflammatory conditions to create a diet plan that supports joint health.

By implementing these arthritis-friendly cooking tips, you can make meal preparation more accessible and enjoyable while reducing joint strain and discomfort. Adapt your cooking methods and kitchen environment to suit your specific needs and preferences for a more comfortable cooking experience.

# Conclusion

"Cookbook for Patients with Arthritis" has been a journey of culinary exploration and empowerment. Throughout this book, we've delved into a world where delicious meals and joint-friendly choices harmonize to enhance the lives of individuals battling arthritis.

As we embarked on this culinary odyssey, we began by understanding the complexities of arthritis, unraveling its various types, symptoms, and diagnostic processes. Armed with this knowledge, we ventured into the realm of anti-inflammatory foods, recognizing them not only as ingredients but as allies in the fight against arthritis. We explored the potential of omega-3 fatty acids and the wisdom of limiting or avoiding certain foods to manage inflammation effectively.

Our journey took us deeper into the practical aspects of arthritis-friendly cooking, where we unveiled the secrets of ergonomic kitchen tools, meal preparation tips, and storage and organization methods that can transform the kitchen into a place of comfort and accessibility.

The heart of this book lies in its delicious and nutritious recipes, carefully crafted to soothe joints and tantalize taste buds simultaneously. From the hearty warmth of the Turmeric Chicken Curry to the refreshing simplicity of the Pineapple and Spinach Smoothie, these recipes cater to the unique needs of arthritis patients without compromising on flavor or variety.

We've shared kitchen wisdom for preparing meals that nurture your joints while celebrating the joy of food. From the moment you pick up a knife or turn on the stove, we've strived to make your culinary journey a delightful and pain-free experience.

But this book is more than just a collection of recipes and cooking tips; it's a testament to resilience and the power of nutrition to enhance the quality of life. It's a reminder that living with arthritis doesn't mean sacrificing the pleasure of savoring a delectable meal.

As we reach the end of this gastronomic expedition, I hope you've discovered not only new recipes but also a newfound confidence in the kitchen. May the flavors and nourishment within these pages inspire you to embrace cooking as a form of self-care, a way to nurture your body, and a source of comfort and joy.

In closing, "Cookbook for Patients with Arthritis" is a celebration of the fusion between culinary creativity and arthritis management. It's a journey that encourages you to savor the moments, cherish your well-being, and relish the artistry of cooking. May each meal you prepare become a small triumph over arthritis, a step toward a more vibrant and flavorful life.